The Indigenous Medicinal Plant Species and their medicinal Uses
Of
Darjeeling and Sikkim Himalaya

By
Sibdas Baskey
Binoy Raj Sharma
Tezoshi khawas

1

Content

37.	*Cucurbita pepo* Linn.	41
38.	*Bombax malabaricum* DC	42
39.	*Dactylicapnos scandens* (D.Don) Hutch.	43
40.	*Daphne cannabina* Wall.	44
41.	*Carica papaya* Linn	45
42.	*Luffa acutangula* Roxb.	46
43.	*Acacia concinna* DC.	47
44.	*Zanthoxylum acanthopodium* DC	48
45.	*Colocasia esculenta* (L.) Schott.	49
46.	*Cynodon dactylon* Linn,	50
47.	*Leea robusta* (Burm. f.) Merr.	51
48.	*Alstonia Scholaris* Br.	52
49.	*Dillenia indica* Linn	53
50.	*Lens culinaris* Linn	54
51.	*Citrus medica* Linn	55
52.	*Ficus religiosa* Linn.	56
53.	*Phyllanthus emblica* Linn.	57
54.	*Adhatoda vasica* Nees.	58
55.	*Lycopersicon esculentum* Will.	59
56.	*Morus indica* Linn.	60
57.	*Delima scandens* Burkill.	61
58.	*Curcuma longa* Linn	62
59.	*Allium cepa* L	63
60.	*Ipomoea batatas* Linn.	64
61.	*Madhuca butyracea* Roxb.	65
62.	*Trachelo spermum fragraus* Hook	66
63.	*Celastrus paniculatus* Willd	67
64.	*Costus speciosus* Smith.	68
65.	*Swertia chirayita* (Roxb. ex Fleming) H. Karst.	69
66.	*Zinziber officinale* Rosc.	70
67.	*Rubia cordifolia* Linn.	71
68.	*Rubus molucannus* Linn.	72
69.	*Cedrela toona* Roxb.	73
70.	*Helianthus annus* Linn.	74
71.	*Cucumis sativus* Linn.	75
72.	*Curcuma aromatic* Salish.	76
73.	*Cydonia oblonga* Will.	77
74.	*Evodia fraxinifolia* Hook.	78
75.	*Abies webbiana* Lind.	79
76.	*Viscum album* Linn.	80

Rhododenron arboreum Sm.

Rhododendon arboreum (Tree Rhododendron) is also commonly known as Lali (Red) gurans in Neplai language and Etok koong in Lepcha language. It belongs to family Ericaceae. It is an evergreen shrub or small tree which grows to the height of 12m (39ft) and produces flowers from April to May. It is recognised for bright red flowers and abundantly distributed in Sikkim and Darjeeling Himalaya region at an altitude ranges from 1500 - 3600 metres.

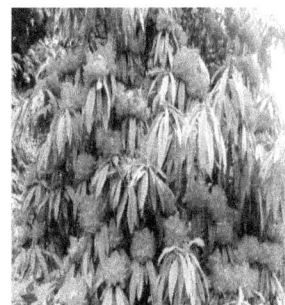

Parts used for medicine
Flowers and petals, young leaves and bark.

Medicinal uses
The young leaves are astringent and poultice. They are made into a paste and then applied to the forehead in the treatment of headaches. The juice of the bark is used in the treatment of coughs, diarrhoea and dysentery. A decoction of the flowers is used to check the vomiting tendency, especially if there is also a loss of appetite. The juice of the flowers is used in the treatment of menstrual disorders. Petals are eaten to assist the removal of any animal bones that have become stuck in the throat. Fresh or dried petals of flower are effective against treatment of dysentery and diarrhoea.

Other uses of the herb:
The juice of the leaves is spread over cots and beds to get rid of bed lice. It can also be used for making charcoal and for fuel. The wood is widely used in Darjeeling and Sikkim for making household implements, building small houses and fences. Planks of the wood are carved to make boxes, cupboards and other furniture. It is a very good fuel, burning well with a long-lasting heat. The excessive collection of its wood for fuel from its natural habitat, and also for making charcoal, has become a cause for conservation concern.

Known hazards of Rhododendron arboreum:
The leaves are poisonous. The flowers can cause intoxication in large quantities.

Allium sativum Linn

Allium cepa is also known by Piyaz in Nepali language and Oo Tsong in Lepcha language. It belongs to the family Alliaceae. It is evergreen biennial bulbous plant grows up to a height of 60 cm and produce flowers during June – July. It is grown widely in the region as vegetable.

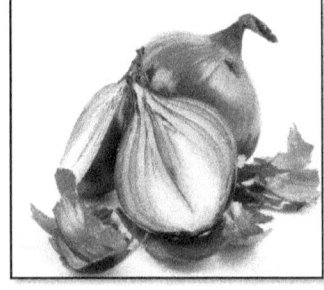

Parts used for medicine
Bulb

Medicinal uses
Although used rarely as a medicinal herb, the onion has a wide range of beneficial actions on human health and when taken (especially raw) on a regular basis will promote the general health of the body. The bulb is anthelmintic, anti-inflammatory, antiseptic, antispasmodic, carminative, diuretic, expectorant, febrifuge, hypoglycaemic, hypotensive, lithontripic, stomachic and tonic. When it is used regularly in the diet it offsets tendencies towards angina, arteriosclerosis and heart attack. It is also useful in preventing oral infection and tooth decay. Baked onions can be used as a poultice to remove pus from sores. The fresh onion juice is very useful as first aid treatment for bee and wasp stings, bites, grazes or fungal skin complaints. The warmed juice can be dropped into the ear to treat earache. It also aids the formation of scar tissue on wounds and thus speeds-up the healing process, and has been used as a cosmetic to remove freckles. Bulbs of red cultivars harvested in mature stage in summer months can be used in homeopathic medicines for the treatment of running eyes and nose.

Other uses of the herb:
The juice of the plant is used as a moth repellent to ward of snakes, scorpions and can also be rubbed onto the skin to repel insects. The juice can also be used as a rust preventive agent on metals and as polishing materials for copper and glass. Onion juice rubbed into the skin is said to promote the growth of hair and remedy for baldness. It is also used as a cosmetic to get rid of freckles. The growing plant is said to repel insects and moles. A spray solution made by boiling 1kg of chopped unpeeled onions in sufficient water is said to increase the resistance of many plants species against diseases and parasites.

Known hazards of *Allium cepa*:
There are cases of poisoning caused by consumption Onion in large quantities to humans and to some mammals. Dogs seem to be particularly very susceptible to this Plant.

Coriandum sativum . L.

Coriandum sativum is known by Dhania in Nepali language and by Oo Su among the Lepcha tribe. It belongs to the family Umbelliferae. It is an annual herb grown over entire Himalayan region. As it has strong aroma it is used in garnishing the various recipes. The flowers on the branches are clustered and are slightly purple in colour. The roots are also important in terms of their aroma and culinary use. The stem can have length up to 3 feet tall.

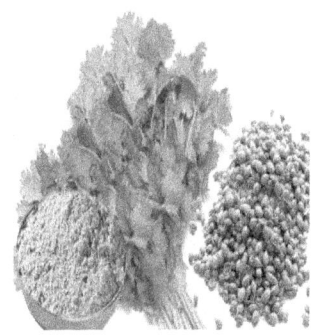

Parts used for medicine
Leaves and seeds

Medicinal uses
Coriander has nutritional value as well as medicinal properties. Its seed contains Iron, Magnesium, Vitamins A, B, and C. Besides, it also contains essential oils like Lenoleic acid, Ascorbic acid, Palmitic acid, Oleic acid, Stearic acid. The presence of monoterpenoid-linalool in Coriander plant helps in curing the problems like bed cold, seasonal fever, nausea, vomiting, stomach disorders as household medicine and also used as a drug against indigestion, worms, rheumatism and pain in the joints.

Other uses of the herb:

Its leaves and seeds are used in culinary, preparation of chutney, salads for its aroma and flavour.

Known hazards of *Coriandum sativum:*

If consumed excessively may cause some of dysfunctional conditions of human body, damage to the liver functions due to the extraordinary volatile constituents. The essential oil components that are found to activate the functioning of liver and certain antioxidants that are usually helpful in treating liver disorders can work reversely if taken excessively as the elements that activate the liver may over emphasize the liver to secret bile and hence producing abnormal conditions. The excessive use of herb is usually not suggested during pregnancy and lactation because of effect of the vital components on the gland secretion that may lead to any abnormal activity of the reproductive gland causing damage to mother or the developing foetus. Prolonged and excessive use of *Coriandrum sativum* can cause breathing problems including tightness of throat and dry throat.

Mentha arvensis Linn.

Mentha arvensis Linn. is known by pudina in Nepali language and Oosoodaong in Lepcha language. This perennial herb belongs to the family Labiatae which grows up to a height of 45 cm. It flowers during May to October. It is cultivated in swampy and marshy areas of Sikkim and Darjeeling Himalayan region.

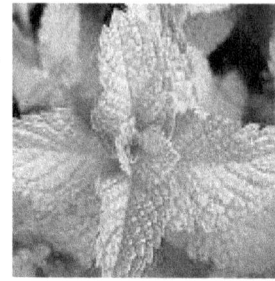

Parts used for medicine
Leaves and tender shoots

Medicinal uses
It is often used as a domestic herbal remedy, being valued especially for its antiseptic properties and its beneficial effect on the digestion. The whole plant is anaesthetic, antiphlogistic, antispasmodic, antiseptic, aromatic, carminative, diaphoretic, emmenagogue, galactofuge, refrigerant, stimulant and stomachic. A tea made from the leaves has traditionally been used in the treatment of fevers, headaches, digestive disorders and various minor ailments.

Other uses of the herb:

The plant is used as an insect repellent. Rats and mice intensely dislike the smell of mint. The plant was therefore used in homes as a strewing herb and has also been spread in granaries to keep the rodents off the grain. The leaves also repel various insects. The sub-species *M. arvensis piperascens* produces the best oil, which can be used as a substitute for, or adulterant of, peppermint oil. Yields of up to 1.6% have been obtained from this sub-species.

Known hazards of *Mentha arvensis*:

Although no records of toxicity have been observed for this species, large quantities of some members of this genus, especially when taken in the form of the extracted essential oil, can cause abortions.

Mimosa pudica Linn.

Mimosa pudica Linn. Is known by Buhari jhar in Nepali language and Aa ook Mook in Lepcha language. It belongs to the family Fabaceae and grows wild in Sikkim and Darjeeling Himalayan region. Stem is erect in young plants, but becomes creeping or trailing with age. The stem is slender, branching, and sparsely to densely prickly, growing 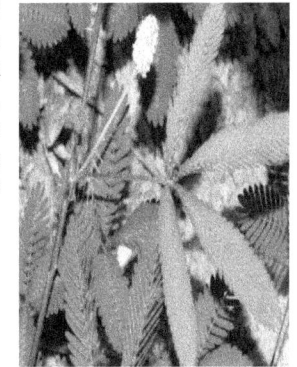 to a length of 1.5 m (5 ft). The *Mimosa pudica* posesses compound leaves.

Parts used for medicine
Whole plant, leaves, and roots.

Medicinal uses
M. pudica is known to possess sedative, emetic, and tonic properties, and has been used traditionally in the treatment of various problems including alopecia, diarrhoea, dysentery, insomnia, tumor and various urogenital infections. Native people of Sikkim and Darjeeling hills use its paste to cure piles.

Other uses of the *Mimosa Pudica*:
Not yet Known

Known hazards of *Mimosa pudica*:
All parts of the *Mimosa pudica* plant are reported to be toxic if taken directly.

Lantana Camara Linn.

Lantana Camara is known by banmara in nepali language and Kadaorip in Lepcha language. It belongs to the family Verbenaceae. It is widely distributed in the Sikkim and Darjeeling Himalaya region and because of its bushy nature it is used as live fencing materials by the native peoples.

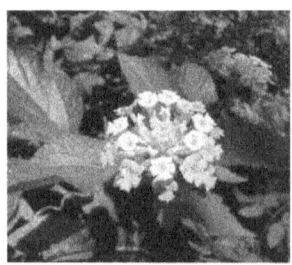

Parts used for medicine
Leaves

Medicinal uses
Lantana camara leaves are boiled and applied against swellings and pain of the body. Its bark is astringent and used as a lotion in cutiginous eruptions, leprous ulcers. Alkaloidal fractions obtained from leaves have been found to lower blood pressure, accelerate deep respiration and stimulate intestinal movements in animals.

Other uses of the shrub
Not yet Known

Known hazards of *L. Camara*
The toxicity occurs only on the consumption of high amount of plants material. It is reported that sheep, cattle and goats are susceptible to lantadenes A, B, D and icterogenic acid toxicity, where as horses, rats, neonatal calves and lambs are not susceptible to lantadene A.

Citrus aurantifolia Christum.

Citrus aurantifolia Christum. is known by nimbu or kagati in
Nepali language and Kachya Koong in Lepcha language. It
belongs to the family rutaceae. *C. aurantiifolia* is a shrubby
tree grows up to 4 to 5 m (16 ft) with many thorns.

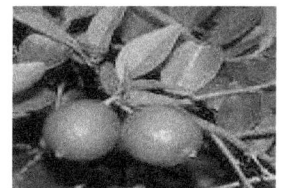

Parts used for medicine
Fruit and tender leaves

Medicinal uses
Its juice has a high content of vitamin C, calcium, potassium and essential oils. It has antiscorbutic,
detoxifying, diuretic, expectorant and antiseptic properties. It avoids fatigue, rheumatic discomfort
and propensity to colds and infections. The leaves and fruit peel contains essential oils with sedative
and antispasmodic virtues. Native people drink its juice extracted from its roots in empty stomach
to kill worms in stomach. They also use fruit as very good appetizer

Other uses of the plant
Used in making prickles and juice

Known hazards of *C. aurantifolia*
As it contains bisabolene its consumption will cause abortion in pregnant women.

Hordeum vulgare Linn.

Hordeum vulgare is known by Jau in Nepali language and kachyer in Lepcha language. It belongs to family Gramineae. It is an annual plant grows up to height of 100 cm and flowers during June to August. It is widely distributed in Sikkim and Darjeeling up to height of 5,000 ft.

Parts used for medicine
Shoots and grains

Medicinal uses
The shoots are diuretic. The seed sprouts are demulcent, expectorant, galactofuge, lenitive and stomachic and are sometimes abortifacient. They are used in the treatment of dyspepsia caused by cereals, infantile lacto-dyspepsia, and regurgitation of milk and breast distension. The seed is digestive, emollient, nutritive, febrifuge and stomachic. It is taken as a nutritious food or as barley water (an infusion of the germinated seed in water) and is of special use for babies and invalids. Its use is said to reduce excessive lactation. Barley is also used as a poultice for burns and wounds. The germinating seed has a hypoglycaemic effect. Barley bran may have the effect of lowering blood cholesterol levels and preventing bowel cancer.

Other uses of the herb
The stems, after the seed has been harvested, have many uses. They are a source of fibres for making paper, a biomass for fuel etc. They can be shredded and also used as a mulch marerials.

Known hazards of *Hordeum vulgare*
Not yet Known

Datura fistulosa Linn.

Datura fistulosa is Known by daturo in Nepali language and Kajyoo Khyaamoong Maon in Lepcha language. It is a foul-smelling, erect, annual, freely branching herb that forms a bush up to 2 to 5 ft (60 to 150 cm) tall. The leaves have a bitter and nauseating taste and remains even after the leaves have been dried. Generally it flowers during the summer. The fragrant flowers are trumpet-shaped, white to creamy or violet. The fruits are covered by spines when matured. It grows in wild in streams and riversides of Sikkim and Darjeeling Himalayan region.

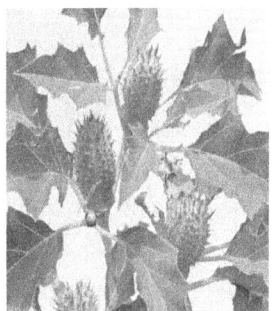

Parts used for medicine
Roots, leaves and stem

Medicinal uses
Roots, Leaves and stem of the datura are useful for rheumatic swelling, lumbago, sciatica and inflammation complaints. In chronic asthmatic fits, seed are used as smoke which reduces asthmatic fits considerably. The seeds are poisonous and will cause death if taken in overdose. It is also taken against mad dog bites. It contains major chemical constituents as Scopalamine, Daturadiol, Hyoscyamine, Fastudine, Allantoin, Niacin, Vitamin C, Tropine, Noratropine, Meteolodine, hyosine, Fastusic acid.

Other uses of the shrub
Not yet Known

Known hazards of Datura
Careful consideration of the toxicity of the plant is required before its use. Its ingestion induces characteristic symptoms. The mouth becomes dry, an intense thirst develops, the vision gets blurred with prominent mydriasis and the heart rate increases. This is followed by hallucinations, delirium, and loss of motor coordination which may ultimately lead to death by respiratory failure.

Bauhinia variegata Linn.

Bauhinia variegate is known by Kachyik Koong in Lepcha language. It belongs to the family Leguminosae. It is a deciduous tree which grows to a height of 12 m (39 feet) and is found in the lower altitude forests of Sikkim and Darjeeling Himalayan region.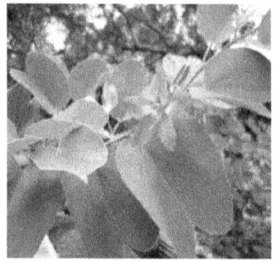

Parts used for medicine
Bark of tree, roots, young leaves, flowers, young buds and fruits

Medicinal uses
The juice of the bark is used in the treatment of amoebic dysentery, diarrhoea and other stomach disorders. A paste of the bark is useful in the treatment of cuts and wounds, skin diseases, scrofula and ulcers inflammation of the joints, skin diseases and diarrhoea. The dried buds are used in the treatment of piles, dysentery, diarrhoea and worms. The juice of the flowers is used to treat diarrhoea, dysentery and other stomach disorders. The root is used as an antidote to snake poison. A decoction of the root is used to treat dyspepsia.

Other uses of the herb
The bark is a source of tannins. It is used for dyeing. Wood is used for house construction and making household implements.

Known hazards of *Bauhinia variegata*
Not yet Known

Amaranthus tricolour Linn.

Amaranthus tricolour is known bathu in Nepali language and Kanyim in lepcha language. It belongs to family Amaranthaceae. It is an annual flowering plant with deep purple flowers. It can grow from 2–3 feet in height and is abundantly grown in Sikkim and Darjeeling region.

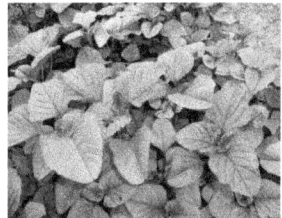

Parts used for medicine
Roots, stem, leaves and seeds

Medicinal uses
It contains protein, fat, carbohydrates, calcium, iron, amarantin, routine, purines, and vitamins (A, B and C). Stem mainly contains linoleic acid and leaves mainly contain amaranthin, linolenic acid, lignoceric acid, arachic acid, spinasterol, monogalactosyldiglyceride, digalactosyldiglyceride, and trigalacto-syldiglyceride. Root are used in the treatment of dysentery, diarrhoea, hemorrhoids, toothache, dermatitis rhus, swelling and pain in scrotum, injuries from falls, metrorrhagia and metrostaxis, leukorrhea. Stem and leaves are used in the treatment of dysentery, infrequent urine and stool, bites by snakes and insects, sores. Seeds are used in the treatment of hordeolum, dark blindness, whitish and turbid urine, hematuria, infrequent urine and stool.

Other uses of the herb
Widely use as vegetable in hills

Known hazards of Amaranthus tricolour
Not yet known

Urtica parviflora Linn.

Urtica parviflora is known by sishnoo in Nepali language and Kazoo in Lepcha language. it belongs to the family Urticaceae. It is a annuals or perennial herbaceous plants, rarely shrubs. They can grow up to height of 10–300 cm depending on the type, location and nutrient status. The perennial species have underground rhizomes. The green parts have stinging hairs. Their often quadrangular stems are unbranched or branched, erect, ascending or spreading. It is widely found in the mid hills of Darjeeling and Sikkim Himalayan region upto the altitudes of 8000 ft.

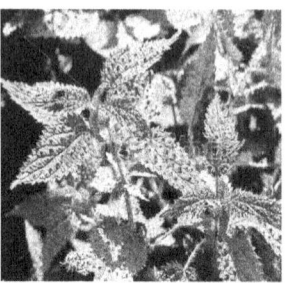

Parts used for medicine
Tender leaves of the plant, roots and flowers

Medicinal uses
Roots are used as medicine for fractures and dislocation, it also helps in delivering babies. After pounding the roots, the juice is taken for the correctiuon of gonorrhoea. Young leaves and flowers are cooked and eaten as vegetables for correction of blood pressure. It helps as a tonic and clearing agent after birth.

Other uses of the herb
A strong flax-like fibre obtained from the stems ca be used in making string, cloth and a good quality paper. It is harvested in early autumn and is retted for fibres. The plant matter left over after the fibres have been extracted are a good source of biomass and have been used in the manufacture of sugar, starch, protein and ethyl alcohol. Its extract is both insect repellent and a good foliar feed to crop plants. If grown as mixed crop with others growing plant increases the essential oil content of other nearby plants, thus making them more resistant to insect pests.

Known hazards of *Urtica parviflora*:
The leaves of the plants have stinging hairs, causing irritation to the skin. This action is neutralized by heat, so the cooked leaves are perfectly safe and nutritious. However, only young leaves should be used because older leaves develop gritty particles called cystoliths which act as an irritant to the kidneys.

Drymaria cordata Linn.

Drymaria is known by abijalo in Nepali language and khaley nayaok in Lepcha language. It belongs to the family Caryophyllaceae. It is a perennial herbs growing up to 0.6 mt. It flowers from July to August. The flowers are hermaphrodite. It grows wild in marshy areas upto 5000 ft. altitudes in the hills of Sikkim and Darjeeling.

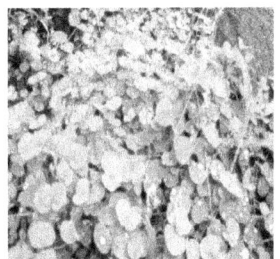

Parts used for medicine
Young tender leaves and shoots.

Medicinal uses
The plant is appetizer, depurative, emollient, febrifuge, laxative and stimulant. The juice of the plant is used for dog and snake bites. Above ground parts can be steamed and smelled during headache and sinus trouble.

Other uses of the herb
Not yet known

Known hazards of *Drymaria cordata*:
Not yet known

Centella asiatica Linn.

Centella asiatica Linn. is known as a Gol patha in nepali language. It belongs to the family Apiaceae and grows in the swampy wetlands areas of Sikkim and Darjeeling hills. The stems are slender, creeping stolons, green to reddish green in color, connecting plants to each other. The leaves are borne on pericladial petioles, around 2 cm. The rootstock consists of rhizomes, growing vertically down. The flowers are white or pinkish to red in color, born in small, rounded bunches (umbels) near the surface of the soil.

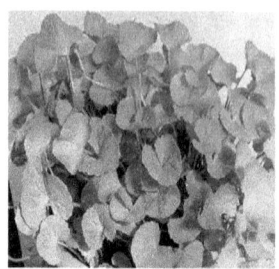

Parts used for medicine
Leaves

Medicinal uses
A part from wound healing, the herb is recommended for the treatment of various skin problems such as leprosy, lupus, varicose ulcers, eczema, psoriasis, diarrhoea, fever, amenorrhea, diseases of the female genitourinary tract and also for relieving anxiety and improving cognition. Triterpenoid, saponins, the primary constituents of Centella asiatica are believed to be responsible for its wide therapeutic actions.

Other uses of the herb
Not yet known

Known hazards of *Centella asiatica*
Not yet known

Rubus ellipticus Sm.

Rubus ellipticus is known by ainselu in Nepali language and kasyum koong in Lepcha language. It belongs to the family Rosaceae. It is evergreen shrub growing wild to the height of 4.5 mt. tall in the open hillsides at an elevations of 1000 - 2600 metres in Himalayas which bears golden yellow fruit.

Parts used for medicine
Root, fruit and tender leaves

Medicinal uses
The plant is astringent and febrifuge. A decoction of the root, combined with *Girardinia diversifolia* root and the bark of *Lagerstroemia parviflora* is used in the treatment of fevers. The root extract is used in the treatment of fevers, gastric troubles, diarrhoea and dysentery. A paste of the roots is applied externally to wounds. Both the roots and the young shoots are considered to be a good treatment for colic pains. The juice of leaf buds combined with *Centella asiatica* and *Cynodon dactylon* are used in the treatment of peptic ulcers. The juice of the fruit is used in the treatment of fever, colic pains, coughs and throat sore. It is a renal tonic and antidiuretic and used in the treatment agaist weakening of the senses, vaginal/seminal discharge, polyuria and micturation during sleep. The roots and young shoots are used in treatment of colic pains and for killing intestinal worms in children.

Other use of *Rubus ellipticus*
A purple to dull blue dye is obtained from the fruit. The plant is grown to conserve soil erosion and is good for soil conservation.

Known hazards of *Rubus ellipticus*
It is advised to wash the fruits properly before eating as it might be made poisonous by snakes as they love drinking water from this plant leaves.

Lyonia ovalifolia Wall.

Lyonia ovalifolia is known by angeri in Nepali language and kaang chyaor koong in Lepcha language. It belongs to family Ericaceae. It is a deciduous shrub which grows up to the height of 2m and flowers during May – June. It prefers sunny situation and grown on hills in scrub and on the edges of oak, pine and rhododendron woods.

Parts used for medicine
Leaves

Medicinal uses
The leaves possess antioxidant and antimicrobial properties and serve as free radicals scavenging as well as natural antibiotic agent. Leaves are used as natural remedy for wounds, cuts and burns. Leaves are crushed and their juices are used externally as an infusion to treat skin diseases and external parasites lice and nits.

Other use of *Lyonia ovalifolia*
Wood is used as a fuel, though is not a very good fuel, and as a charcoal.

Known hazards of *Lyonia ovalifolia*
The young leaves and buds are toxic to goats.

Juglans regia Linn.

Juglans regia is known by okher in Nepali language and kaol koong in Lepcha language. It belongs to family Juglandaceae. It is large, deciduous tree growing up to the heights of 25–35 mt. and trunk up to the diameter 2 mt. It grows wild in the forest of upper, middle and lower hill of Sikkim and Darjeeling.

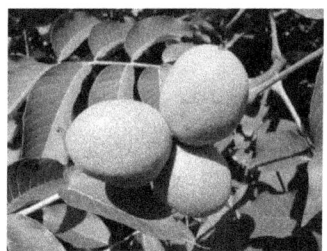

Parts used for medicine
Bark, leaves, fruit

Medicinal uses
Walnut is considered to be an astringent, anti-fungal and antiseptic. Due to its tannin content a decoction of Walnut leaves can be used in treatment of diarrhoea. Walnut oil is used in treatment of tapeworms. A decoction made from the fruit can stimulate the production of thyroid hormones. Usage of nut decoction on a daily basis can thus be beneficial in case of hypothyroidism. Walnut can help in treatment of various skin problems such as acne, eczema, dermatitis, herpes, itching and psoriasis. Walnut can also be very beneficial as a hair care ingredient. It is said that a decoction made from dried leaves could help in prevention of hair fall.

Other Uses of *Juglans regia*
Trunk can be use as timber.

Known hazards of *Juglans regia*
Not yet known

Prunus puddum Roxb.

Prunus Pudum is known by arucha in Nepali language and kaong kee koong in Lepcha language. It belongs to family Rosaceae which is deciduous tree growing to height of 30 mt. It is found in the forests of upper, middle and lower hill of Sikkim and Darjeeling.

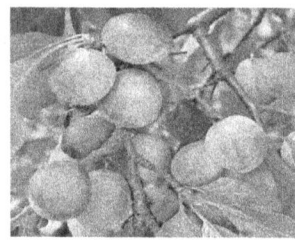

Parts used for medicine
Bark, tender branches and fruit.

Medicinal Uses
The paste made from bark can be applied in healing fracture of bones. It is used in the treatment of stone and gravel in the kidney, bleeding disorders, burning sensation and skin diseases. It is a best anti-abortifacient. The young small branches crushed and soaked in water when taken internally stops abortion.

Other uses of *Prunus puddum*
Used as table fruit as well as wood as fuel

Other Hazards of *Prunus puddum*
Not yet known

Ananas comosus Mar.

Ananas comosus is known by anarash in Nepali language and kaong chyey in Lepcha language. It belongs to family Bromeliaceae. It is a herbaceous perennial which grows to the height of 1.0 to 1.5 mt. tall. Pineapple carries out CAM photosynthesis, fixing carbon dioxide at night and storing it as the acid malate and then releasing it during the day, aiding photosynthesis. It is cultivated in lower foothills of Sikkim and Darjeeling.

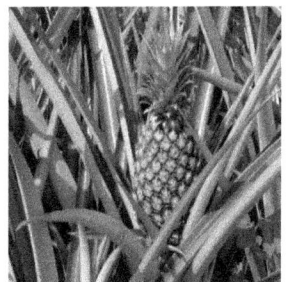

Parts used for medicine
Leaves, Fruit and green fruit

Medicinal Use
Juice is extracted from leaves and taken fresh to treat hiccough and constipation as it has anthelmintic and cholagogue properties. It destroys and expels intestinal worms of the children. Its fruit is digestive, diuretic, laxative, diaphoretic and antiscorbutic and use to treat gastric irritability and jaundice. Juice of the fruit helps to cure swollen and bleeding gums and aids digestion. The fruit is rich in manganese and good for proper bone growth and strengthening bone and connective tissues. Pineapple is also useful for maintaining oral health and helpful in healing process after a dental surgery. Treating colds, throats sore and acute sinusitis are other health benefits of pineapple.

Other uses of *Ananas comosus*
Used as a bio-mass for preparation compost manure.

Other Hazards of *Ananas comosus*
The green fruit can acts as abortifacient, cause abortion if taken in excess amount.

Semecarpus anarcardium Linn.

Semecarpus anarcardium is known by bhalayo in Nepali language and kaong hee koong in Lepcha language. It belongs to family Anacardiaceae. It is a deciduous tree grown wild in the forests of mid and upper hill of Sikkim and Darjeeling.

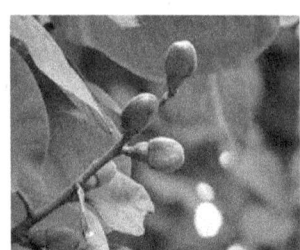

Parts used for medicine
Fruit

Medicinal Uses
Its nuts contain a variety of biologically active compounds such as biflavonoids, phenolic compounds, bhilawanols, minerals, vitamins and amino acids, which show various medicinal properties. The fruit and nut extract shows various activities like anti-atherogenic, anti-inflammatory, antioxidant, antimicrobial, anti-reproductive, CNS stimulant, hypoglycemic, anticarcinogenic and hair growth promoter. The local people use the paste of nuts for treating all kinds of skin diseases.

Other uses of *Semicarpus anarcardium*
Not yet known

Other Hazards of *Semecarpus anarcardium*
The leaves of the plants have hairs causing irritation to the skin.

Piper longum Linn.

Piper longum is known by lamche marich in Nepali language and kuntim paot in Lepcha language. It is a flowering vine belongs to family Piperaceae, cultivated for its fruit, which is usually dried and used as a spice and seasoning. It is grown wild in the forests of lower hill and valleys of Sikkim and Darjeeling region.

Parts used for medicine

Fruits and Roots

Medicinal Uses

Native people use the fruits in treatment of asthma, cough, rheumatism, gonorrhoea, piles and spleen. Roots are used for curing hoarseness .The powdered roots with powdered black pepper taken with milk is good for women for development of breast .Powdered fruits taken with sugar or molasses induces sound sleep. Long pepper is used to improve appetite and digestion, as well as treat stomachache, heartburn, indigestion, intestinal gas, diarrhoea, and cholera. Its other uses includes treatment of headache, toothache, vitamin B1 deficiency (beriberi), coma, epilepsy, fever, stroke, trouble sleeping (insomnia), leprosy, extreme tiredness, enlarged spleen, muscle pain, nasal discharge, paralysis, psoriasis, intestinal worms, snake bites, tetanus, thirst, tuberculosis, and tumors. Women also use Indian long pepper to stimulate menstrual flow and to treat menstrual cramps, infertility, and loss of interest in sexual activity.

Other uses of *Piper longum*

Not yet known

Other Hazards of *Piper longum*

Over consumption causes abortions in pregnant woman.

Stephania hernandifolia Walp.

Stephania hernandifolia is known by tamerkey in Nepali language and kuntek rik in Lepcha language. It belongs to family Menispermaceae. It is a herbaceous perennial vines growing to around four metres tall, with a large, woody caudex used as medicinal plant by herbalists for treating various diseases, one of which is diabetes mellitus, in Darjeeling. It grows wild in the forests and valleys of lower hill of Sikkim and Darjeeling.

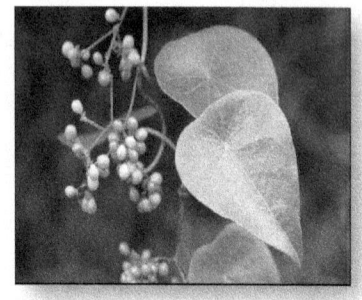

Parts used for medicine
Leaves and roots

Medicinal uses
The plant root is of large globular shape and is bitter in taste and use in the treatment of diabetes, fever, diarrhoea and urinary diseases. It contains alkaloids, carbohydrates, tannins and phenolic compounds , steroids, flavonoids, saponins and lignins. The leaves are used in the spewing of boils.

Other uses of *Stephania hernandifolia*
The young roots are eaten as vegetables.

Other Hazards of *Stephania hernandifolia*
Known to possess antispermatogenic or male infertility effect. The folk women use the crude aqueous extract of leaves for the prevention of pregnancy.

Entanda scandens Benth.

Entanda scandens is known by pangra in Nepali language and koolook paot in Lepcha language. It belongs to the family Fabaceae. The seeds of plant have thick and durable seed coat which allows them to survive for longer periods. It grows wild in the forests and valleys of lower hill of Sikkim and Darjeeling.

Parts used for medicine
Seed and Bark

Medicinal use
Juice of the bark and wood are used for skin diseases. The inner seeds are used for washing hair to clear dandruff. It is poisonous but it can be eaten after removing the poison by certain process. The seeds powder pest on application subsides swollen neck glands. The plant is also used as ointment against jaundice, toothache, ulcers and to treat muscular and skeletal problems.

Other Uses of *Entanda scandens*
The seeds are sought after as pieces of jewelry and as good-luck charms

Other Hazards of *Entanda scandens*
Not yet known

Gynocardia odorata R.Br

Gynocardia odorata is known by bhadarey fal in Nepali langage and took koong in Lepcha language. It belongs to family Achariaceae. The trees grow up to the height of 30 mt. tall. The leaves are glossy, entire, and alternate. The flowers are yellow and sweet-scented. The fruit is round, ash-colored, and when mature averages weight varies from 10 to 20 pounds. It is distributed in the lower hill forests of Sikkim and Darjeeling.

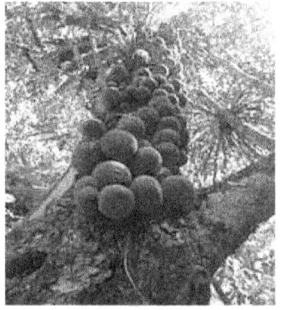

Parts used for medicine
Seeds

Medicinal Uses
Seeds oil is used as a remedy for leprosy, Lupus, Scrofula. It is also used in eczema and other skin diseases and chronic rheumatism, stiffness of joints, ulcers, and various cutaneous eruptions.

Other uses of *Gynocardia odorata*
Tree can be used as timber and fuel.

Other hazards of *Gynocardia odorata*
The oil is eaten after going through certain process otherwise it is poisonous.

Momordica charantia Linn.

Momordica charantia is known by tittey karela in Nepali language and khaaktik in Lepcha language. it belongs to the family cucurbitaceae, which has herbaceous, tendril-bearing vine grows up to 5 mt height. It is widely cultivated in Sikkim and Darjeeling as vegetables.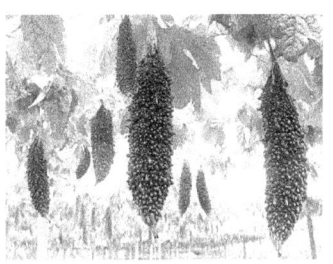

Parts used for medicine
Tender Leaves and fruit

Medicinal uses
The fruit is bitter, cooling, digestible, laxative, antipyretic, anthelmintic, appetizer and used in the treatment of biliousness, blood diseases, anaemia, urinary discharges, asthma, ulcers, bronchitis etc. Juice extracted from the fruit has charantin which acts in reduction the sugar level in diabetic patients. Its leaves extract is used for remedy against burning as it has wound healing properties. Fruits are beneficial in gastric problem. Oil extracted from the seed is used in the treatment of breast cancer.

Other Uses of *Momordica charantia*
Widely consumed as vegetable

Other Hazards of *Momordica charantia*
An excessive consumption result in drastic lowering blood sugar levels in diabetics (Hypoglycemia), which is sometime, is not good. It should not be taken by pregnant women as it can cause bleeding.

Dichroa febrifuga Low.

Dichroa febrifuga is known by Neel kamal in Nepali language and gey boo khaanaok in Lepcha language. It is a shrub belonging to the family Hydrangeaceae. It is abundantly distributed in the forests of upper and middle hill of Sikkim and Darjeeling.

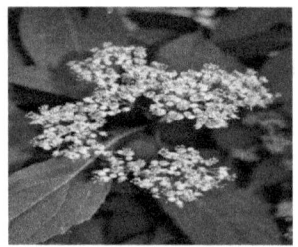

Parts used for medicine
Roots and leaves

Medicinal uses
This leaves are purgative. They are used in the treatment of stomach cancer. Leaf juice is used to treat coughs, colds and bronchitis. A decoction of the stem bark is used in the treatment of fevers. A decoction of the leaves is used to treat malarial fever. The root contains several alkaloids and is emetic, expectorant, febrifuge and purgative. The juice from the root is used in to treat fevers and indigestion. This plant is 26 times more powerful than quinine in the treatment of malaria but causes vomiting. Substances in the plant are 100 times more powerful than quinine, but they are poisonous.

Other uses of *Dichroa febrifuga*
Wood is used as fuel

Other Hazards of *Dichroa febrifuga*
Their excessive uses can causes vomiting and sometimes lethal to human being.

Curcuma caesia Roxb.

Curcuma caesia is known by kalo hardi in Nepali language and gey sying in Lepcha language. *Curcuma caesia* belongs to the family Zingiberaceae. It is a perennial herb with bluish-black rhizome, native to Sikkim and Darjeeling hills. The rhizome of black turmeric has a high economic importance owing to its putative medicinal properties.

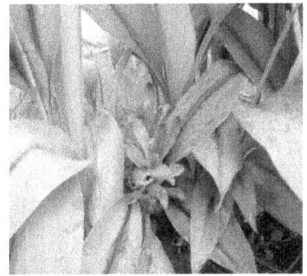

Parts used for medicine
Rhizome

Medicinal uses
Dried rhizomes and leaves of *Curcuma caesia* are used in piles, leprosy, asthma, cancer, wounds, impotency, fertility, tooth ache, vomiting, and allergies. Its rhizome relieves the flatulence. Fresh rhizome decoction is used against diarrhoeia and relief from stomachache. The fresh rhizome paste of *Curcuma caesia* is applied during the snake bite and scorpion bite to detoxify the poison .The rhizome is used for the treatment of cough, fever, dysentery, worm infection. The fresh rhizomes are used in leprosy, cancer, epilepsy, anti-helmenthic, aphrodisiac, gonorrhoreal discharge. Rhizome of *Curcuma caesia* is used in the treatment of rheumatic arthritis. Crushed rhizome paste is applied against cur or injury to control bleeding and quick healing. The rhizome *Curcuma caesia* is administered during inflammation of tonsils. The roots of the *Curcuma caesia* is grounded into powder and used with water to treat gastric disorder.

Other uses of the *Curcuma caesia*
Use in religious activities

Other hazards of *Curcuma caesia*
Not yet known

Michelia champaca Linn.

Michelia champaca is known by chaap in Nepali language and gok rip in Lepcha language. It belongs to Magnoliaceae family. It grows wild in the forests of lower hill of Sikkim and Darjeeling.

Parts used for medicine
Bark, root, root bark, leaves, flowers

Medicinal uses
Plant is deobstruent, bitter, stomachic, emmenagogue, febrifuge and demulcent. Bark is bitter, tomnic, astringemt, antiperiodic and helps to reduce fever and ejects phlegm from the throat and lungs by coughing and spitting. Flower and fruits are also used in nausea and fever, also useful as promoting urine in kidney and in gonorrhoea. Flowers are used as stimulant, tonic, puragative and carminatie, also as demulcent and diuretic. A decoction of the flowers is effective in case of dyspepsia, nausea and fevers. It is also useful in preventing scalding in gonorrhoea and renal ounces.

Other uses of *Michelia champaca*
Not yet known

Other Hazards of *Michelia champaca*
Not yet known

Flemingia congesta Roxb.

Flemingia congesta is known by bhatte in Nepali language and nyeepit mook in Lepcha language. It belongs to the family Fabaceae. It is a erect legumineous shrub widely distributed in lower and middle hills of Darjeeling and Sikkim Himalayan region.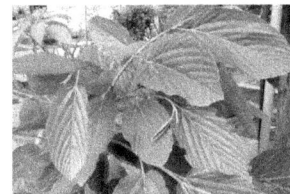

Parts used for medicine
Leaves and Bark

Medicinal Uses
The paste prepared from the leaves and barks is used for external application against ulcers and swellings. Fresh root juice has anti-bacterial properties and used against treatment of endema.

Other uses of *Flemingia congesta*
Not yet known

Other hazards of *Flemingia condesta*
Not yet known

Luffa acutangula Roxb.

Luffa acutangula is known by ghiraula in Nepali language and taryaa bee in Lepcha language. It belongs to the family cucurbitaceae. It grows as a flowering annual vine with pollinated flowers developing into cylindrical green fruits filled with seeds in a system of manyintertwined cellulose fibres. It is cultivated throughout Sikkim and Darjeeling hills as vegetable.

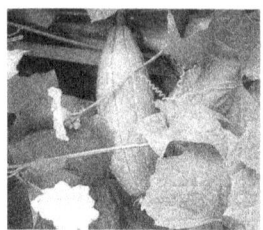

Parts used for medicine
Seed and Leaves

Medicinal Uses
The fruit is edible especially when young and it contains group of compounds such as phenolics, lavonoids, oleanolic acid, ascorbic acid, a-tocopherol, carotenoids, chlorophylls, triterpenoids and ribosome-inactivating proteins, which makes it highly effective when used for medicinal purpose. It has antitumour and antiviral activities, and also induce uterine contraction to hasten child birth. Seeds are used as purgative. The juice of leaves is dropped into the eyes in granular conjunctivitis.

Other uses of *Luffa acutangula*
Use as vegetable and matured fruit as sponge for taking bath.

Other hazards of *Luff actungula*
Not yet known

Shorea robusta Gaertn.

Shorea robusta is known by sakhwa in Nepali language and tuk tal koong in Lepcha language. It belongs to the family Dipterocarpaceae. Moderate to slow growing tree and can attain heights of 30 to 35 mt. height and a trunk diameter of up to 2-2.5 mt. It is very good timber tree and grows wildly in the forest of lower hill of Sikkim and Darjeeling.

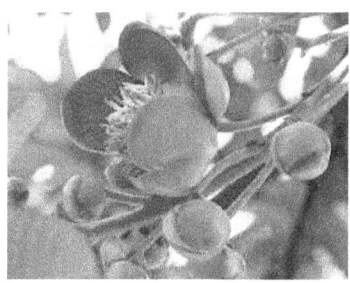

Parts used for medicine
Resins and leaves
Medicnal uses
Resin is composed for chemicals like hydroxyanone, dammarenediol II, Ursolic acid etc. The resin is astringent and aphrodisiac, detergent and is used in dysentery and for fremigation. The resin burnt over the fire gives out thick volumes of fragrant smoke, and it is much used for fumigating rooms occupied by the sick. It also repels mosquitoes and other insects. Its resin along with honey or sugar is given in dysentery and bleeding piles problem. It is also used in the treatment of gonorrhoea and for weak digestion. Its bark decoction is used as drops in ear problems. Besides, its fruits are also used in diarrhoea.

Other uses of *Shorea robusta*
Not yet known
Other hazards of *Shorea robusta*
Not yet known

Albizia julibrissin Durazz.

Albizia julibrissin is known by siris in Nepali language and tuk chyer koong in Lepcha language. It belongs to family fabaceae. It is a small deciduous tree growing to 5–16 mt. tall with a broad crown of level or arching branches. The bark is dark greenish grey in colour and striped vertically as it gets older. It grows wild in the forests of lower and mid hill of Sikkim and Darjeeling.

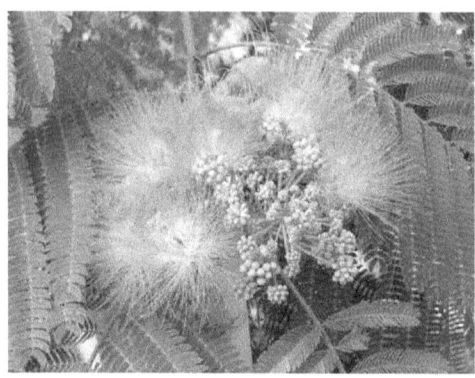

Parts used for medicine
Bark and seed

Medicinal uses
The flower heads are carminative, digestive, sedative and tonic. They are used internally in the treatment of insomnia, irritability, breathlessness and poor memory. The flowers are harvested as they open and are dried for later use. The stem bark is anodyne, anthelmintic, carminative, discutient, diuretic, oxytocic, sedative, stimulant, tonic, vermifuge and vulnerary. It is used internally in the treatment of insomnia, irritability, boils and carbuncles. Externally, it is applied to injuries and swellings. The bark is harvested in spring or late summer and is dried for later use. A gummy extract obtained from the plant is used as a plaster for abscesses, boils etc and also as a retentive in fractures and sprains. Bark and seeds are given in piles and diarrhoea problems. The Powdered root bark is used to strengthen gums of teeth. Juice of the younger leaves are put in the eyes against the problem of blindness.

Other uses of *Albizia julibrissin*
A gummy extract of the plant is used as a plaster. No more details are given. Wood are used for furniture, industrial applications, firewood etc.

Other hazards of *Albizia julibrissin*
Not yet known

Artemisia vulgaris Linn.

Artimisia vulgaris is known by titeypati in Nepali language and tuknyil in Lepcha language. It belongs to the family Asteraceae. It is a tall herbaceous perennial plant growing 1–2 mt. tall with a woody root. It grows wild in the forests of mid and lower hill of Sikkim and Darjeeling.

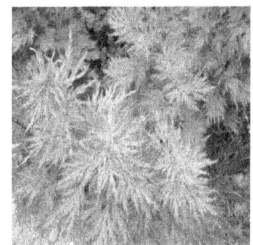

Parts used for medicine
Whole plant

Medicinal uses
Whole plants and leaves are rubbed externally in skin diseases and ulcers. In nose bleeding crushed leaves is and used to block the nostrils for stopping bleeding. Leaf extract in boiled water is used in treatment of gout and rheumatism. The young shoots are boiled and eaten to increase appetite and promotes digestion. The whole plants are burnt over the fire to repel the mosquitoes and other insects through its smoke. The floors are rubbed with its leaves to drives away insects as fleas etc. It is also used in cleaning or purifying in religious ceremonies. It is very effective in curing malaria and ordinary fever. Mugwort has a long history of using it in herbal medicine especially in matters connected to the digestive system, menstrual complaints and the treatment of worms. All parts of the plant are anthelmintic, antiseptic, antispasmodic, carminative, cholagogue, diaphoretic, digestive, emmenagogue, expectorant, nervine, purgative, stimulant, slightly tonic and used in the treatment of women's complaints. The leaves are also said to be appetizer, diuretic, haemostatic and stomachic. They can be used internally or externally. An infusion of the leaves and flowering tops is used in the treatment of nervous and spasmodic affections, sterility, functional bleeding of the uterus, dysmenorrhoea, asthma and diseases of the brain. The leaves have an antibacterial action, inhibiting the growth of Staphylococcus aureus, Bacillus typhi, B. dysenteriae, streptococci, E. coli, B. subtilis, Pseudomonas etc. The leaves are harvested in August and can be dried for later use. The stem is also said to be antirheumatic, antispasmodic, and stomachic. The roots are tonic and antispasmodic. They are said to be one of the best stomachics. They are harvested in the autumn and dried for later use. The leaves placed inside the shoes are said to be soothing for feet sore. The compressed dried leaves and stems are used in moxibustion.

Other uses of *Artimisia vulgaris*
The fresh or the dried plant repels insects so it can be used as a spray against crop insect-pests but caution is advised since it can also inhibit plant growth. A weak tea made from the infused plant is a all-purpose good insecticide. An essential oil from the plant kills insect larvae. The down on the leaves makes good tinder for starting fires.

Other hazards of *Artimisia vulgaris*
It is slightly toxic and should never be used by pregnant women especially in their first trimester, since it can cause a miscarriage. Large prolonged dosage can damage the nervous system.

Paederia foetida Linn

Paderia foetida is known by tulpitrik in lepcha language. It belongs to the family Rubiaceae. It is very bad smelling creeper and grows wild in the lower regions of Sikkim and Darjeeling.

Parts used for medicine

Leaf, root and fruits

Medicinal uses

Roots are considered to be emetic, emollient and carminative and useful in colic, spasm, rheumatism and gout. Leaves and roots are considered to be a tonic that stimulates the central nervous system. Alleviates spasms and anticancer (leaf), immunosuppressive and antiinflammatory (plant). It contains active ingredients like Paederoside, asperoloside and scandoside (stem and leaf), beta-sitosterol, friedelan and epifriedelinol (plant). Young leaves and shoots are cooked and eaten as it is considered wholesome and nutritive for the sick and convalescent. Its juice is taken as well as rubbed over the body for rheumatic cure. The juice of the leaves is also given to children in diarrhoea. The fruit is pounded and smeared on the teeth against toothache and decay but it turns the tooth black. It can be used against Hemorrhoids, in piles, inflammation of spleen, liver and chest pain (root), as a tonic (root and leaf), in rheumatism (plant), as poultice to relieve distension of abdomen due to flatulence and also used in herpes (leaves) to children in diarrhoea (leaf juice) and for vesical calculi (leaf decoction).

Other uses of the *Paderia foetida*

Not yet known

Other hazards of *Paderia foetida*

Not yet known

Mussaenda frondosa Linn

Mussaenda frondosa is known by dhobiphul in Nepali language and tumbaar rik in Lepcha language. it belongs to the family Rubiaceae. It is a small shrub of 1.5 to 2 mt. tall and 1.5 to 2 mt. width and found in the forests of lower hill of Sikkim and Darjeeling.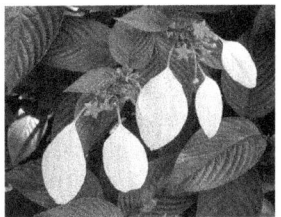

Parts used for medicine
Flower, root

Medicinal uses
The flowers contain anthocyanins, hyperin, quercetin, rutin, ferulic, sinapic acids, beta-sitosterol glucoside and has diuretic, antiasthmatic, antiperiodic properties. The whole plant of is used to cure cough, bronchitis, fever, wounds, ulcers, leucoderma, pruritus and its leaves makes a excellent herbal shampoo. The flowers are used against asthma problem and the juice of the roots is used as remedy for jaundice. It can be applied externally for the cure of skin eruptions, ulcers etc. Root is used in the treatment of white leprosy.

Other uses of the *Mussaenda frondosa*
Not yet known

Other hazards of *Mussaenda frondosa*
Not yet known

Amonum subalatum Roxb.

Amomum subalatum is known by thulo alichi in Nepali language and Tung barp in Lepcha language. It belongs to the family Zingiberaceae. Plant grows up to 4 mt. in length in thick clumps and starts bearing its prized seed pods soon after about two years age of plantation. Each pod measures about 1-2 cm in length. It is widely cultivated Sikkim and Darjeeling hills.

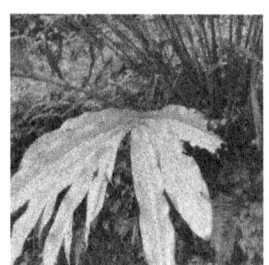

Parts used for medicine
Seeds and roots

Medicinal uses
The therapeutic properties of cardamom oil have been reported in many traditional medicines. Cardamom-oil have found its application in many traditional medicines as antiseptic, antispasmodic, carminative, digestive, diuretic, expectorant, stimulant, stomachic ,tonic and as local anesthetic, antioxidant in addition to health promoting and disease preventing roles. The decoction of cardamom is used as gargle in infection of teeth and gums. It is also used in treatment of gonorrhoea. Roots is pounded and given to the cattle for curing urine haemorrhage. Cardamom is a good source of minerals like potassium, calcium, and magnesium, riboflavin, niacin, vitamin-C.

Other uses of *Amomum subulatum*
Use as spice for its aroma and flavour.

Other hazards of *Amomum subulatum*
Avoid pods that appear light and that are with surface discoloration or spots, which may feature mould (fungal infection).

Cucurbita pepo Linn.

Cucurbita pepo is known by farsi in Nepali language and tung zaong in Lepcha language. It belongs to the family Cucurbitaceae. Pumpkin plant is an annual, herbaceous creeper. It has a flexible climbing stem and large dark-green leaves. Leaves are heart-shaped with well marked nerves and slightly hairy. Flowers are orange and trumpet-shaped. Fruits are oval to spherical and green or orange in colour. It is grown widely by the people of Sikkim and Darjeeling as vegetable.

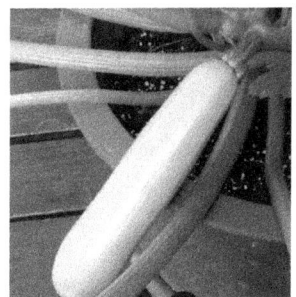

Parts used for medicine
Seeds and pulp

Medicinal uses
Pumpkin acts as demulcent, diuretic, nervine, and taenifuge. Traditionally Pumpkin was used to treat kidney problems and intestinal parasites. It has a good laxative and diuretic property. It has shown to be helpful in treatment of initial prostate hyperplasia problem. If used externally its pulp is an excellent emollient, reducing dryness of skin. It is useful in treatments of pimples, spots, freckles and burns. Pumpkin plant also acts as a good immune booster containing great amount of vitamins A, C and glycine. It is a gentle and safe remedy for a number of complaints, especially as an effective tapeworm remover for children and pregnant women for whom stronger medicines are unsuitable. The seeds are mildly diuretic and vermifuge. The complete seed together with the husk is used to remove tapeworms. The seed is ground into fine flour then made into an emulsion with water and eaten to expel the tapeworms or other parasites from the body. The seed is used to treat hypertrophy of the prostate. The seed is high in zinc and has been used successfully in the treatment of early stages of prostate problems. The diuretic action has been used in the treatment of nephritis and other problems of the urinary system. The leaves are applied externally against burns. The fruit pulp is used as a decoction to relieve intestinal inflammation.

Other uses of *Cucurbita pepo*
Seed oil is used for lighting.

Other hazards of *Cucurbita Pepo*
If matured Pumpkin is eaten as vegetable by pregnant woman it causes abortion.

Bombax malabaricum DC

Bombax malabaricum is known by tungloo koong in Lepcha language. It belongs to the family Malvaceae. It is a tree used in Ayurvedic traditional medicine to treat many ailments and health conditions. It is a very large tree and grows up to a height of 40 mt. and are spiny when young and with buttresses when mature. It grows wild in the forests of lower hill and valleys of Sikkim and Darjeeling.

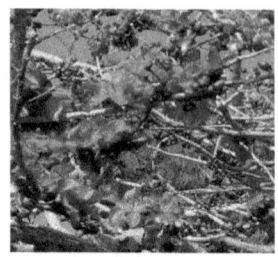

Parts used for medicine
Young shoots, resins and gum.

Medicinal uses
It has anti-helicobacter, diuretic, anthelmitic, vermifuge, vermicide, antimicrobial and antioxidant properties. It is use in treatment of inflammatory conditions, diarrhoea, fever, chronic inflammation, catarrhal affection. The gum like juice is used in dysentery. Young roots are used in gonorrhoea problem. The resin is used for arousing sexual desire. Anthelmintic effects of it help the body to expel helminths or parasitic worms.

Other uses of *Bombax malabaricum*
Not yet known

Other hazards of *Bombax malabaricum*
Not yet known

Dactylicapnos scandens (D.Don) Hutch.

It is known as thol in Lepcha language. It is a smaller plant found in the forests of middle and upper hill of Sikkim and Darjeeling.It belongs to family Papaveraceae.It is herbaceous climbing perennial herbs, about 3-5 m long. Stems slender, angular, grooved, glabrous. Leaves 2 or 3 times ternately compound, exstipulate, about 5 cm long, petiole about 2.5-3 cm long, leaflets ovate-spathulate to ovate-elliptic, about 1-3.5 x 0.5-2 cm across, base acute to cuneate usually unequal, margin entire, apex acute to obtuse with mucronate tip, terminal leaflet larger than the lateral leaflets, lateral veins about 5-7 either side of the midrib, first or lowest pair almost near the base, petiolules slender, grooved, about 0.5-1 cm long,

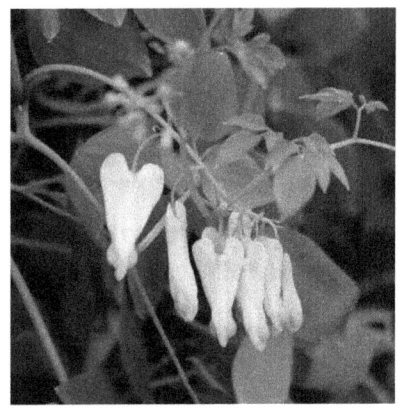

Parts used for medicine
Roots

Medicinal uses
The juice extracted from the roots is used for stopping overflow of menstruation.

Other uses of *Dicetra thalictrifolia*
Not yet known

Other hazards of *Dicentra thalictrifolia*
Not yet known

Daphne cannabina Wall.

Daphne cannabina is known by dyeynaok koong in Lepcha language. It belongs to family Thymelaeaceae. It is evergreen scented shrub which can grow up to height of 2 mt. and flowers during January to April. The plant grows wild in the forests of upper hill of Sikkim and Darjeeling.

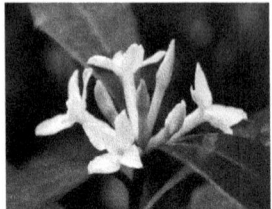

Parts used for medicine

Roots

Medicinal uses

The juice of the roots combined with molasses is used in the treatment of fevers and intestinal problems. A decoction of the bark is used to treat fevers. The powdered seeds are anthelmintic. Roots are used as antidotes in poisoning. Drinking the extract of the roots causes diarrhoea and vomiting which ultimately cleans out the poison from the body of affected person.

Other uses of *Daphne cannabina*

Very good quality paper is made from the inner bark. It is one of the main sources of handmade paper. The fibre in the inner bark can be used to make rope.

Other hazards of *Daphne Cannabina*

All parts of the plant are poisonous. Skin contact with the sap can cause dermatitis in some people.

Carica papaya Linn

Carica papaya is known by mewa in Nepali language and naaroo paot in Lepcha language. It belongs to the family Caricaceae. It is cultivated all over Sikkim and Darjeeling up to the elevation of 4000 ft.

Parts used for medicine
Leaves, fruit, seed, latex

Medicinal uses
It has therapeutic properties as analgesic, amebicide, antibiotic, antibacterial, cardiotonic, cholagogue, digestive, emmenagogue, febrifuge, hypotensive, laxative, pectoral, stomachic, vermifuge. It is used in the treatment of warts, cancers, tumors, corns, and indurations of the skin. The extract from the root is used in the treatment of tumors of the uterus, piles, jaundice and yaws and reduce urine acidity in humans. latex is used in the treatment of psoriasis, ringworm, and prescribed for the removal of cancerous growths. The fruit, leaves, latex and seeds are used to treat skin diseases, indigestion, enlargement of liver and spleen, worms, diseases of heart, cough and fever. The fruit eaten either raw or ripe keeps the enhances the digestive power.

Other uses of *Carica papaya*
Use as fruit.

Other hazards of *Carica papaya*
Externally the latex is irritant, dermatogenic, and vescicant. If somebody intakes the latex it causes severe gastritis. Some people are allergic to the pollen, the fruit, and the latex. Papain can induce asthma and rhinitis. The acrid fresh latex can cause severe conjunctivitis and vesication. If a pregnant woman takes the milky liquid of this raw fruit it causes abortion.

Luffa acutangula Roxb.

Luffa acutangula is known by zinganey in Nepali language and taryaa bee in Lepcha language. It belongs to the family cucurbitaceae. It is cultivated widely throughout Sikkim and Darjeeling hills as vegetable.

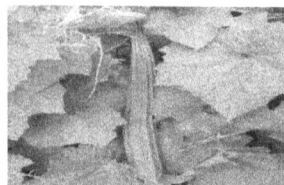

Parts used for medicine
Fruit, Seed and roots

Medicinal Uses
It is a nutritive vegetable with fibers, vitamins and minerals. It contains low calories and fats. It is used against the treatment of jaundice. Seeds are used as purgative. The juice of leaves is dropped into the eyes in granular conjunctivitis. Ridge gourd has blood purifying properties and also clears the pimples and acne problems. It helps in the purification, restoration and nourishment of the liver and is also helpful in the liver detoxification resulting from alcohol intoxication. Cellulose fibers helps in the treatment of constipation and also effective in the treatment of piles. Chemicals like insulin, alkaloids and charantin helps in maintaining cholesterol, blood sugar and urine sugar levels. Roots has diuretic properties and when added to milk or water are helpful in the removal of kidney stones. The leaves are useful in the treatment of dysentery. The leaves are also good when used as dressing in the diseases such as inflammation of spleen, ringworms, piles and even leprosy. Pounded leaves mixed with garlic are applied locally for relief in leprosy.

Other uses of *Luffa acutangula*
Sponge has been used traditionally as an exfoliating product while bathing.

Other hazards of *Luff actungula*
Not yet known.

Acacia concinna DC.

Acacia concinna is known by naangaa maanyee paot in Lepcha language. It belongs to the family Fabaceae. It is a climbing shrub found throughout the tropical forest. The fruit is known in India as shikaka

Parts used for medicine

Leaves, pods and bark

Medicinal uses

The plant extracts are used in natural shampoos or hair powders. The bark contains high levels of saponins which is foaming agents and is found in several other plant species used as shampoos or soaps. The Saponin containing plants have a long history of use as mild cleaning agents. Saponins from the plant's pods have been traditionally used as a detergent. Leaves are used as purgative and against bile and liver trouble.

Other uses of *Acacia concinna*

Not yet known

Other hazards of *Acacia cocinna*

Not yet known

Zanthoxylum acanthopodium DC

Zanthoxylum acanthopodium is known by naong ryoo paot in lepcha language. It belongs to the family Rutaceae. It is found in the lower hills of Sikkim and Darjeeling. It is also found southern China (western Guangxi Guizhou, Sichuan, Tibet Autonomous Region, and Yunnan), Bangladesh, Bhutan, northern India (Arunachal Pradesh, Assam, Manipur, Meghalaya, Mizoram, Nagaland, Sikkim, Uttar Pradesh, and West Bengal), Nepal, Laos, Burma, northern Thailand Vietnam, Indonesia (northern Sumatran highlands), and Peninsular Malaysia.

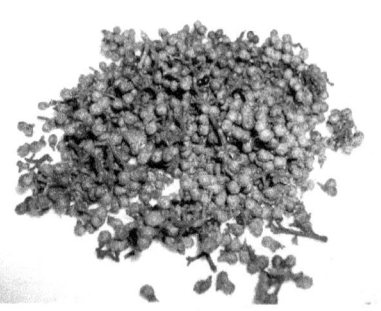

Parts used for medicine
Seeds and Bark

Medicinal Uses
Seeds and Bark are used as an aromatic tonic in fever, dyspepsia and cholera. Distilled arrack of the fruit is applied on the affected parts to cure the gout and rheumatism. It is also used as remedy for the toothache.

Other uses of *Zanthoxylum acanthopodium*
the seed pericarps are used as spices in cooking

Other hazards of *Zanthoxylum acanthopodium*
Not yet known

Colocasia esculenta (L.) Schott.

Colocasia esculenta is known by many in Nepali language and pazaok luktuk in Lepcha language. *Colocasia esculenta* is a herbaceous perennial plant belonging to the Araceae family. The leaves are also used as leafy vegetables. The large green leaves are often described as 'elephant ear' and they can grow up to the height of 1-2 mt.

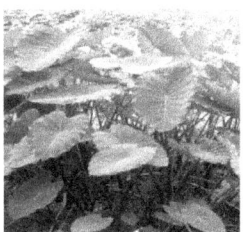

Parts used for medicine
Leaves and root

Medicinal uses
Leaf contains phenols, tannin, saponins, steroids, quinine, trepenoids, glycosides, alkaloids except flavonoids. The leaf juice has antibacterial activity against scorpion sting or snake bite as well as it is used against food poisoning of plant origin. Its roots are pounded and cooked in butter and eaten as medicine for curing Tuberculosis, Typhoid, Pneumonia, Otitis, Urinary tract infection and Diarrhoea.

Other uses of *Colocasia esculenta*
Use as leafy vegetable.

Other hazards of *Colocasia esculenta*
Not yet known.

Cynodon dactylon Linn,

Cynodon dactylon is known by dhoobo in Nepali language and paong pook in Lepcha language. It belongs to the family Gramineae. It is a evergreen perennial herb found everywhere in Sikkim and Darjeeling hill. It is a valuable grass for fodder and soil conservation due to its long runners that roots at the nodes. It is also used in religious ceremony of Hindu Nepali community.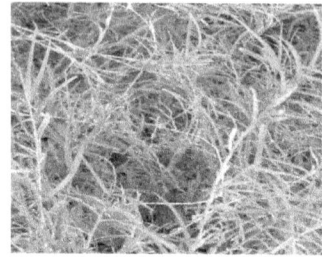

Parts used for medicine
Leaves, roots and tender stem.

Medicinal uses
It is anabolic, antiseptic, aperients, astringent, cyanogenetic, demulcent, depurative, diuretic, emollient, sudorific, and vulnerary. A decoction of the root is used as a diuretic in the treatment of dropsy. An infusion of the root is used to stop bleeding from piles. The juice of the plant is astringent and is applied externally to fresh cuts and wounds. It is used in the treatment of chronic diarrhoea and dysentery. It is also useful in the treatment of catarrhal ophthalmia. The juice is also used in the treatment of dropsy and anasarca. The leaf juice has also been used in the treatment of hysteria, epilepsy and insanity. The plant is traditionally used as remedy for anasarca, calculus, cancer, carbuncles, convulsions, cough, cramps, cystitis, diarrhoea, dropsy, dysentery, epilepsy, headache, haemorrhage, hypertension, hysteria, insanity, kidneys, laxative, measles, rubella, snakebite, sores, stones, tumours, uro-genital disorders, warts, and wounds. Decoction of roots is beneficial in dropsy and in secondary syphilis. Crushed roots are used in chronic gonorrhoea. It is also useful in inflammation of the eye membranes or external structure.

Other uses of *Cynodon dactylon*
Use as fodder and soil conservation agent due to its long runners that covers the soil surface.

Other hazards of *Cynodon dactylon*
Not yet known.

Leea robusta (Burm. f.) Merr.

Leea robusta is known by pun tom in lepcha language. It belongs to the family Vitaceae. It is found at the stream side of Sikkim and Darjeeling hills.

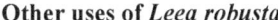

Parts used for medicine
Leaves, young shoots and roots

Medicinal uses
Root tubers are red in colour, mucilaginous and astringent. It is externally used as anodyne and internally against diarrhoea. Leaves and young shoots are baked in fire and bandaged over the fractured or sprained part gives relives from pain and cures it. The vapour of boiling plant relives the body ache and also helps in subsiding the swollen legs. It cures the wounds sores, ringworm and gunieaworm.

Other uses of *Leea robusta*
Not yet known.

Other hazards of *Leea robusta*
Not yet known.

Alstonia Scholaris Br.

Alstonia Scholaris is known by pur vok koong in lepcha language. It belongs to the family Apocynaceae. It is a large evergreen tree grows almost to the height of 25 mt. Its milky juice is bitter taste. It has a dark grey bark with whorled branches. It grows wild in the forests of mid and upper hill of Sikkim and Darjeeling.

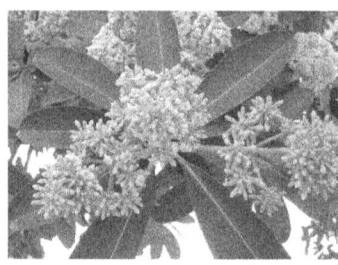

Parts used for medicine
Milky exudates, leaves as well as the bark and roots.

Medicinal uses
The bark contains alkaloids like ditamine and ditain. It Purifies the blood and cures the respiratory disorders. It rejuvenates the digestive system. It is a cytotoxic herb which is used to stop the cancerous growths. It is also useful in curing fevers and skin ailments. The tree has been used as an astringent in ayurvedic medical science for centuries. It is known for its astringent like properties. The tonic made from this tree is used as a febrifuge, anti choleric, vulneray and emmenagogue. The bark is useful in skin diseases and rheumatism. The juice of the root when taken with milk cures leprosy. The bark powder after drying can be mixed with pig's food increases the body very fast.

Other uses of *Alstonia Scholaris*
Not yet known.

Other hazards of *Alstonia Scholaris*
Not yet known.

Dillenia indica Linn

Dillenia indica is known by phaamsyee koong in Lepcha language. It belongs to the family Dilleniaceae. It grows wild in the forests of mid and upper hill of Sikkim and Darjeeling.

Parts used for medicine
Root, fruit, young leaves and bark.

Medicinal uses
Root is used to cure food poisoning. Paste of root and bark is applied externally to cure sprains. Young bark and leaf is good astringent. Fruit juice when mixed with water and sugar forms a cooling drink given against fever and cough. Ripe fruit juice removes flatulence, improves semen quantity and combats weakness. Bark and leaves are used to stop discharge of blood.

Other uses of *Dillenia indica*
Not yet known.

Other hazards of *Dillenia indica*
Not yet known.

Lens culinaris Linn

Lens culinaris is known by fyetlaasyee in Lepcha language. It belongs to the family Fabaceae. *Lens culinaris* is a annual plants growing to the height of 0.5 mt. It is found in the lower regions of Sikkim and Darjeeling.

Parts used for medicine
Seed and seed pod

Medicinal uses
The seeds are mucilaginous and laxative. They are considered to be useful in the treatment of constipation and other intestinal problems. The paste made from seed and seed pods are useful in cleansing application in foul and indolent ulcers. The extract of seed or grains after boiling cures measles.

Other uses of *Lens culinaris*
Not yet known.

Other hazards of *Lens culinaris*
Not yet known.

Citrus medica Linn

Citrus medica is known by bimira in Nepali language and beesu paot in Lepcha language. It belongs to the family Rutaceae. It is a slow growing shrub or small tree grows to the height of 4.5 mt. with stiff branches and twigs and spines in the leaf axils. Fruit is oblong, oval, narrowing toward the top. Its skin is thick, fleshy and very aromatic. It grows wild in the forests of lower hill of Sikkim and Darjeeling.

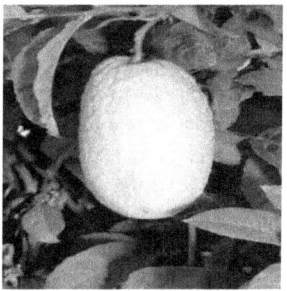

Parts used for medicine
Fruits, leaves & seeds.

Medicinal uses
Citrus medica is rich in citric acid, sulphuric acid, glucose, volatile oils, potassium, calcium, Vitamin C. It is used as herbal remedy for pulmonary and intestinal disorders and halitosis. It is use as herbal remedy for diarrhoea. It aids digestion, eliminates gastric acidity, stimulates functioning of the liver. It is also helpful in cases of flatulence and vomiting. It is used in the treatment of in headach especially in migrain. The rind is dried and use against dysentery.

Other uses of *Citrus medica*
The fruit is used to make pickle and the plant is a good root stock against some diseases of cultivated citrus species.

Other hazards of *Citrus medica*
Some herbs could react with certain medication. Therefore, it is advisable to consult your doctor before consumption of any herb.

Ficus religiosa Linn.

Ficus religiosa is known by nebhara in Nepali language and baor koong in Lepcha language. It belongs to the family Moraceae. It is a large dry season deciduous or semi-evergreen tree grows up to the height of 30 mt. tall and with a trunk diameter of about 3 mt. *F. religiosa* has a religious significance in the tribal community. It grows in the forests of lower and mid hill of Sikkim and Darjeeling.

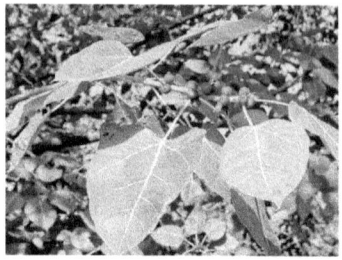

Parts used for medicine
Bark, roots, buds, leaves, fruits and latex.

Medicinal uses
In traditional medicine various parts such as stem bark, root bark, aerial roots, vegetative buds, leaves, fruits and latex are used in diabetes, vomiting, burns, gynaecological problems, dysentery, diarrhoea, nervous disorders, tonic and astringent. Phytochemical investigation of plant's barks showed the presence tannins, saponins, flavonoids, steroids, terpenoids and cardiac glycosides. Bark is powdered and is taken in gonorrhoea. The leaves and young shoots are taken as purgative. The fruits are also eaten.

Other uses of *Ficus religiosa*
It is a good fodder plant.

Other hazards of *Ficus religiosa*
Not yet known.

Phyllanthus emblica Linn.

Phyllanthus emblica is known by amala in Nepali language and braong paot in Lepcha language. It belongs to the family is Phyllanthaceae. It is a small or medium sized deciduous tree that has spreading branches. The trunk of the tree is crooked and has a smooth exfoliating bark. The digitate compound leaves are light green in colour and are closely set near the branch. They are usually 10 to 15 mm long and 3 to 8 mm wide. It is widely distributed in Sikkim and Darjeeling regions.

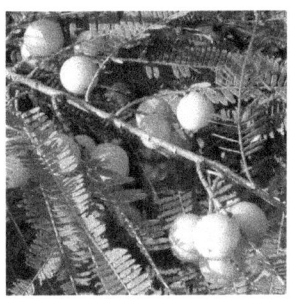

Parts used for medicine
Leaves, seeds, root, bark, fruit and flowers

Medicinal uses
The *Phyllanthus emblica* is rich in polyphenols like gallic acid, phyllemblic acid and ellgic acid. It also contains a large amount of ascorbic acid, cytokinins and fatty acids like behenic. Its fruit pulp contains protein, calcium, magnesium, iron, phosphorus and reducing sugars. Bark and fruits are used in diarrhoea and dysentery. It also helps in digestion of food. Fresh juice of the fruit mixed with milk or honey is good in gonorrhoea. When the juice of the fruit is taken with pure butter and honey it cures obstinate hiccough. Juice is taken with honey to cure white leucorrhoea in woman. The Juice is beneficial in reliving the pain in the urine trouble and brings sensation to the vagina.

Other uses of *Phyllanthus emblica*
Fruit is used as pickle

Other hazards of *Phyllanthus emblica*
Not yet known

Adhatoda vasica Nees.

Adhatoda vasica is known by boosyeekaa in Lepcha language. It belongs to the family Acanthaceae. This is an evergreen perennial shrub having leathery leaves. The flowers are dense and large having large bracts and whitish pink/purple coloured. The plant is often grown as a hedge and its leaves and twigs are utilized as green manure. It grows wild in the lower hilly areas of Sikkim and Darjeeling.

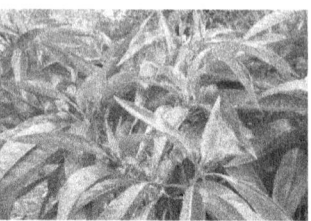

Parts used for medicine
Whole plant or its roots, leaves, bark and flowers

Medicinal uses
It contain alkaloids, triterpenes and phytosterols, flavonoids and essential oils. Roots, barks, leaves and flowers help to remove phlegm, bile and impurities of blood. It is also used against cough, asthma, fever, vomiting, gonorrhoea, leprosy and tuberculosis. Flowers are use in gonorrhoea. Leaves are valuable antiseptic. Flowers are eaten as vegetables. The rhizomes and leaves are used to treat cold and cough, anthrax, abscesses, asthma and, jaundice, urticaria, tuberculosis, scabies, haematuria, pneumonia and throat infection.

Other uses of *Adhatoda vasica*
Not yet known

Other hazards of *Adhatoda vasica*
The plant should be avoided during pregnancy except at the time of birth since it contains oxytocic which stimulates utrine-contractions and abortifacient which induces abortion. Avoid consuming excessive doses of adhatoda since it can cause irritation in the alimentary canal, vomiting or diarrhoea.

Lycopersicon esculentum Will.

Lycopersicon esculentum is known by rumbera in Nepali language and byooroo paot in Lepcha language. It belongs to the family Solanaceae. The plants grow to the height of 1–3 mt. and have a weak stem that often sprawls over the ground and over other plants. It is a perennial in its native habitat, although often grown in temperate climates as an annual.

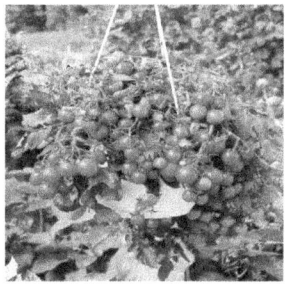

Parts used for medicine
Fruits and root

Medicinal uses
A sliced fruit is used as treatment for burns, scalds and sunburn. Its pulp shows good result against oily skin. Decoction of root is effective in treatment of toothache. Tomato skin contains lycopine, a substance that prevents heart attacks. Lycopine also avoids prostate problems and urine disorders. Fruits are very rich in vitamin A and C.

Other uses of *Lycopersicon esculentum*
Plant used as insects repellent and effective and poisonous insecticide against ants. Oil from the semi-dried seed used in soap making.

Other hazards of *Lycopersicon esculentum*
All green parts of the plant if consumed raw is poisonous.

Morus indica Linn.

Morus indica is known by kimbu in Nepali language and mikraap koong in Lepcha language. It belongs to the family Moraceae. Mulberry tree is deciduous tree which grows up to the height of 7.5 mt. and bears sweet flavoured fruits. It grows wild in the forest of lower hills of Sikkim and Darjeeling.

Parts used for medicine
Bark and fruit

Medicinal uses
The fruit is aromatic, cooling and laxative. It is used in the treatment of fevers. The bark is anthelmintic and purgative. A paste of the bark is used in the treatment of gingivitis. The root is anthelmintic and astringent. A decoction of root is used in the treatment of internal parasites. The decoction of the leaves is used as a gargle in inflammation of the vocal cord and for curing a hoarse voice and infections of the mouth and throat. Roots leaves and fruits of mulberry helps to control blood sugar, diabetes, food poisoning, tape worm, and reduce cholesterol.

Other uses of *Morus indica*
It is rearing plant of Silk worm

Other hazards of *Morus indica*
Not yet known

Delima scandens Burkill.

Delima scandens is known by mungkyo rik in Lepcha language. It belongs to the family Dilleniaceae. It is evergreen woody climber which grows in the forests of lower and mid hills of Sikkim and Darjeeling.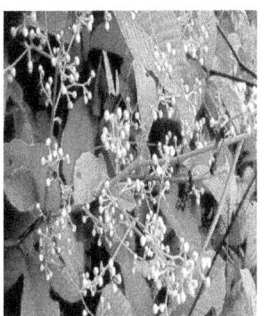

Parts used for medicine
Leaves & roots

Medicinal uses
A decoction of the plant is given in dysentery and coughs. Leaves are used for the treatment of boils. Root acts as astringent and used as external application for burns.

Other uses of *Delima scandens*
Not yet known

Other hazards of *Delima scandens*
Not yet known

Curcuma longa Linn

Curcuma longa is known by hardi in Nepali language and mung gaa in Lepcha language. It belongs to the family Zingiberaceae. It is an herbaceous perennial plants which grows to a height of 60 -90 cm. Flowers of the turmeric appear on a spike like the stalk. Its flowers are sterile and do not produce viable seed. The lamina is green in colour on upper surface and pale green below and it is 30 -40 cm long and 8 -12 cm wide. It is cultivated all over Sikkim and Darjeeling hills for domestic uses.

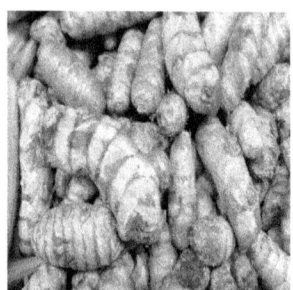

Parts used for medicine
Rhizomes
Medicinal uses
The rhizome powders applied over cuts, bruises, or scrape stops bleedig as well as heal the wounds with antiseptic effect. Decoction of rhizome is taken as remedy for cough and cold. The fresh juice is used as anti-parasitic for skin infections. It is taken as the blood purifier and is very useful in the common cold, leprosy, intermittent, affections of the liver, dropsy, inflammation and wound healing. The rhizome of the turmeric plant is highly aromatic and antiseptic. It is even used for contraception, swelling, insect stings, wounds, whooping cough, inflammation, internal injuries, pimples, injuries, as a skin tonic. Milk boiled with the turmeric is the good remedy for cold and cough. It is given in liver ailments and jaundice.

Other uses of *Curculna longa*
Used as spices for colouring curry.
Other hazards of *Curculna longa*
Not yet known

Allium cepa L

Allium cepa is known by piyaj in Nepali language and mung goo in Lepcha language. It belongs to the family Alliaceae. It is extensively cultivated all over Sikkim and Darjeeling hills.

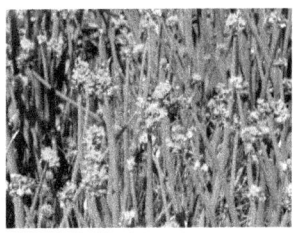

Parts used for medicine
Bulb

Medicinal uses
It is eaten raw on a regular basis for better health of the body. The bulb is anthelmintic, anti-inflammatory, antiseptic, antispasmodic, carminative, diuretic, expectorant, febrifuge, hypoglycaemic, hypotensive, lithontripic, stomachic and tonic. When used regularly in diet it offsets tendencies of angina, arteriosclerosis and heart attack. It is also useful in preventing oral infection and tooth decay. Baked onions can be used as a poultice to remove pus from sores. Fresh onion juice is a very useful first aid treatment for bee and wasp stings, bites, grazes or fungal skin complaints. It also aids the formation of scar tissue on wounds, thus speeds up the healing process and has used as a cosmetic to remove freckles. Bulbs of red cultivars are harvested when mature in the summer and used to make a homeopathic medicine. It is used particularly in the treatment of running eyes and nose.

Other uses of *Allium cepa*
The juice of the plant is used as a moth repellent and can also be rubbed onto the skin to repel insects. The plant juice can be used to rust prevent on metals and as a polish for copper and glass. Onion juice rubbed into the skin is said to promote the growth of hair. It is also used as a cosmetic to get rid of freckles. The growing plant is said to repel insects and moles. A spray made by pouring enough boiling water to cover 1kg of chopped unpeeled onions is said to increase the resistance of other plants to diseases and parasites.

Other hazards of *Allium cepa*
Not yet known

Ipomoea batatas Linn.

Ipomoea batatas is known by sakarkhanda in Nepali language and byooroo paot in Lepcha language. It belongs to the family convolvulaceae. It is widely cultivated in Sikkim and Darjeeling hills for food.

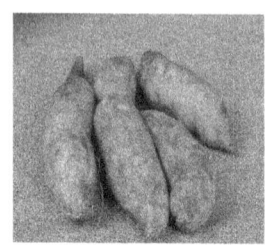

Parts used for medicine
Tubers
Medicinal uses
Ipomoea batatas is an extremely versatile and delicious vegetable that possesses high nutritional value. It is also a valuable medicinal plant having anti-cancer, antidiabetic, and anti-inflammatory activities. Its root is laxative and good source of starch.

Other uses of *Ipomoea batatas*
Not yet known
Other hazards of *Ipomoea batatas*
Not yet known

Madhuca butyracea (Roxb.) J.F.Macbr.

Madhuca butyracea is known by churi in Nepali language and yel paot in Lepcha language. It belongs to the family Sapotaceae. It is a large deciduous tree that grows up to the height of 20mt. tall with dark gey or brownish bark. It grows wild in the forests of lower and mid hill of Sikkim and Darjeeling.

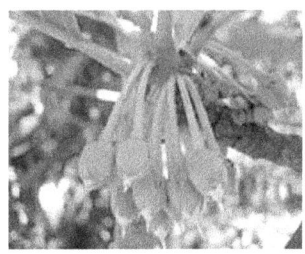

Parts used for medicine
Fruit & seed

Medicinal uses
Seed fat is applied against headache, rheumatism, boils and pimples. It is also used as mollient for chapped hands and feet in winter. Juice of the bark is used for the treatment of indigestion, asthma, rheumatism and boils and also as anthelmintic. Juicy pulp of ripe fruit is eaten fresh. The extract from the seed is used as an ointment for rheumatism. It is also used to soften the dry skin of hands, legs and face which often cracks in winter.

Other uses of *Madhuca butyracea*
Some people use it as hair oil and raw material for soap. Bark and oil cake are used as fish poison. Oil cake is also used as fertilizer to protect crops from harmful insects and worms

Other hazards of *Madhuca butyracea*
Not yet known

Trachelo spermum fragraus Hook

Trachelo spermum fragraus is known by duudhi in Nepali language and yaok chyaon rik in Lepcha language. It belongs to the family Apocynaceae. It is an evergreen woody plant growing to the height of 3 mt. It is found in the forests of lower and mid hills of Sikkim and Darjeeling.

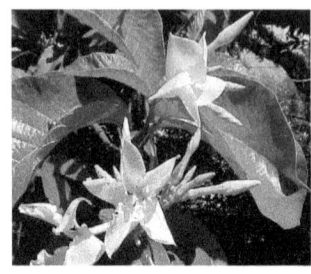

Parts used for medicine

Bark & leaves

Medicinal uses

The bark is bitter in taste and used in preparation of tonic to treat against malaria. It is also useful in diarrhoea and dysentery. Its milky juice is applied to ulcers. The leaves stem and twigs are used for treating rheumatic arthritis, nervous disorders, and urine retention and as a tonic against weak muscles or nerves.

Other uses of *Trachelo spermum fragraus*

Not yet known

Other hazards of *Madhuca butyracea*

Not yet known

Celastrus paniculatus Willd

Celastrus paniculata is known by ruklim in
Lepcha language. It belongs to the family
Celastraceae. It grows wild in the forest of lower
hill of Sikkim and Darjeeling.

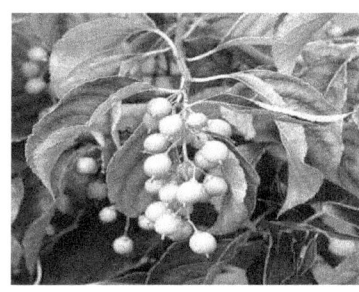

Parts used for medicine

Medicinal uses
Seeds are used in the treatment of rheumatism,
paralysis and leprosy. Seeds are made into paste
and applied to cure scabies. One seed, if taken daily for a month will cure lumbago and
rheumatism.

Other uses of *Celastrus paniculata*
Not yet known.
Other hazards of *Celastrus paniculata*
Not yet known.

Costus speciosus Smith.

Costus speciosus is known by betlauri in Nepali language. It belongs to the family Zingiberaceae. It is an erect plant grows up to the height of 2.7 mt. with tuberous root stock and sub-woody stem at the base. It is found in swamps and marshy places up to the altitudes of 5,000 ft in Sikkim and Darjeeling hills.

Parts used for medicine
Rhizome

Medicinal uses
Rhizomes extraction has tigogenin and diosgenin which is bitter, astringent, acrid, cooling, aphrodisiac, purgative, anthelmintic, depurative, febrifuge, expectorant and tonic and useful in burning sensation, constipation, leprosy, worm infection, skin diseases, fever, asthma, bronchitis, inflammations and anaemia. The rhizomes are used in several diseases with mixture of honey. It cures eczema and bowel complaints. Rhizome has been used to treat fever, rash, asthma, bronchitis, and intestinal worms.

Other uses of *Costus speciosus*
Not yet known.
Other hazards of *Costus speciosus*
Not yet known.

Swertia chirayita (Roxb. ex Fleming) H. Karst.

Swertia chiryata is known by chiroto in Nepali language. It belongs to the family Gentianaceae. The plant is an erect annual herb with branching, cylindrical and robust stems. Leaves are lurid with greenish yellow and purple tinge on lower leaf surface and stem. Its seeds are smooth and have many angle.

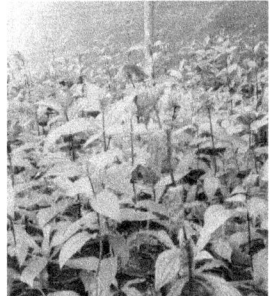

Parts used for medicine
Whole plant

Medicinal uses
Chirata contains chiratin and amarogentin which is an effective drug for reducing fevers especially in malarial fever. It is also effective in hysteria and convulsion. The herb strengthens stomach and promotes the digestive actions. It is good for treatment of dyspepsia and diarrhoea. It also contains anthelmintic which destroys intestinal worms and parasites. The root of the plant is useful in checking hiccups and vomiting. The herb as well as its extracts is used in several skin problems. It is much used in urinary complaints with uneasiness in the region of the kidneys, frequent urging to urinate, and in cases of uric acid deposits. In addition, this bitter tonic is also said to be effective in protecting functional activity of liver. It is laxative and an appetizer. It is a bitter tonic and when taken with white sandalwood paste it stops internal haemorrhage of stomach.

Other uses of *Swertia chirata*
Not yet known.

Other hazards of *Swertia chirata*
Chirata make ulcers in the intestine and excess dose has risk of developing hearing problems.

Zinziber officinale Rose.

Zinziber officinale is known by aduwa in Nepali language and heng in Lepcha language. It belongs to the family Zingiberaceae. It is an herbaceous perennial plants which grows annual stems about a meter tall bearing narrow green leaves and yellow flowers known for strong aroma and flavour. It is cultivated throughout the hills of Sikkim and Darjeeling for centuries.

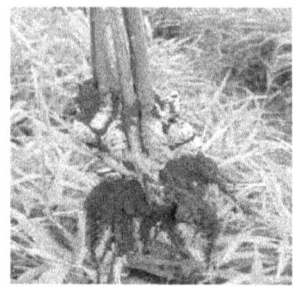

Parts used for medicine
Rhizome

Medicinal uses
Ginger is an old herbal medicine good for different ailments, abdominal bloating, cough, diarrhoea, rheumatism. According to the Tibetan medicine it is consider to be helpful in treatment of various inflammatory joint diseases. Ginger relives different forms of nausea and vomiting problems, motion and morning sickness and problems with indigestion. Ginger is also considered helpful in treatments of headaches, menstrual pain, throat sore, fevers and ulcerative colitis. Some gastrointestinal problems, such as gases and heartburn can also be treated with Ginger. Rhizome is used for fever and goitre. It is a valuable medicine for asthma palpitation, piles and dropsy. When eaten with butter cure rheumatism. The juice of ginger and turmeric taken with honey cure cold, asthma and when mixed with lemon juice cures dyspepsia. Powder of dried ginger applied on the forehead with boiled water cures headache.

Other uses of *Zinziber officinale*
Prickles and candies.

Other hazards of *Zinziber officinale*
Taken in excessive dose will cause light diarrhoea and burning sensation in stomach.

Rubia cordifolia Linn.

Rubia cordifolia is known by vyumrik in Lepcha language. It belongs to the family Rubiaceae. It is a climbing or scrambling herb with red rhizomatous base and roots. It is found in the forests of upper hills of Sikkim and Darjeeling.

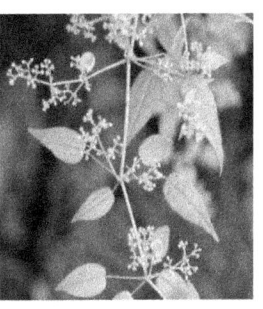

Parts used for medicine
Roots fruit and leaves

Medicinal uses
Powdered dried roots and fruits are taken internally for the treatment of skin diseases and disorders of spleen. It is also used for the treatment of burns, bone fractures and dysentery. It is also taken as tonic, antitussive and useful in chronic low fevers. Decoction from roots is prescribed to cure jaundice, paralytic affections, urinary troubles, amenorrhea and to the mother after delivery for cleansing and shrinking of the uterus. The root decoction is effective to regulate menstruation cycles and other troubles of women. The root extracts of *R. cordifolia* has astringent, themogenic, febrifuge, antidysenteric, antihelmintic, galactopurifier, ophthalmic, and rejuvenating effect. It is used to cure tuberculosis and intestinal ulcer. Roots and a fruit made into paste and is used as an ointment in skin disease.

Other uses of *Rubia cordifolia*
The roots and leaves give a dye for colouring wool blankets, carpets, clothes etc.

Other hazards of *Rubia cordifolia*
Not yet known.

Rubus molucannus Linn.

Rubus molucannus is known by safok jyu in Lepcha language. It is a deciduous shrub belongs to the family Rosaceae. It is climbing, straggling, prickly shrub, reaching to a height of 2 to 3 mt. with branches covered by wooly hairs. It is found in the forests and valleys of lower hill of Sikkim and Darjeeling.

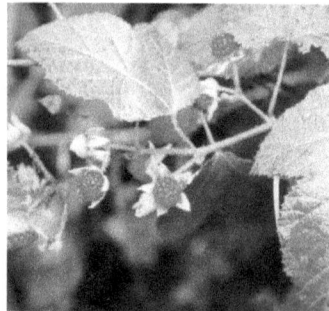

Parts used for medicine
Leaves, fruits and root

Medicinal uses
The leaves are abortifacient, astringent and emmenagogue. The fruit is considered to be a useful remedy for the nocturnal micturation of children (bed-wetting). Root, leaves, and fruit are used for diarrhoea. Root decoction is used for dysentery. The leaves are used as antihypertensive. Heated leaves are applied to the abdomen against abdominal pain. Leaves are useful for promoting the menstrual discharge.

Other uses of *Rubus molucannus*
Fruit yields a purple dye.

Other hazards of *Rubus molucannus*
Not yet known.

Cedrela toona Roxb.

Cedrela toona is known by tooni in Nepali language and samaal koong in Lepcha language. It is a forest tree belongs to the family Meliaceae. It grow to the height of 60 metres. and its trunk can reach up to 3 mt. in girth. It is found in the forests of lower, mid and upper hill of Sikkim and Darjeeling.

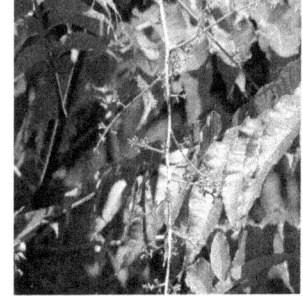

Parts used for medicine
Bark & flower.

Medicinal uses
Decoction of bark is astringent, carminative, febrifuge, ophthalmic and styptic and used for cleaning wounds and curing various forms of ulceration. Powder of the bark is considered antiseptic and is dusted over gangrenous ulcers. Decoction of flowers is used as an antispasmodic. The flowers are used for promoting the menstrual discharge. A decoction is used in the treatment of diarrhoea, chronic dysentery, flatulence, bloody stools, seminal emissions, leucorrhoea, metrorrhagia and gonorrhoea.

Other uses of *Cedrela toona*
Used in the manufacture of decorative applications such panelling, joinery and furniture.

Other hazards of *Cedrela toona*
Not yet known.

Helianthus annus Linn.

Helianthus annus is known by ghaam phool in Nepali language and satsuk rip in Lepcha language. It is an annual crop growing up to the height of 4.6 mt. tall. It is known for its edible oil and edible fruits. It belongs to the family Asteraceae. It is cultivated in gardens as showy flowers all over the hill of Sikkim and Darjeeling.

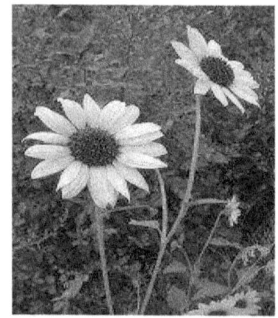

Parts used for medicine
Seed

Medicinal uses
Sunflower seeds have antioxidant, anti-inflammatory, diuretic and expectorant properties. They are helpful in reducing symptoms of asthma, osteoarthritis and rheumatoid arthritis and help in cases of bronchial, pulmonary and laryngeal problems. They can be applied as an addition to therapy of colon cancer, high blood pressure and migraine headaches. It has good amount of magnesium content. Sunflower seeds can also act as prevention against heart attacks and strokes. Sunflower leaves can be used as an infusion to treat high fevers, lung problems and diarrhoea. As a poultice sunflower root is used against snake and spider bites.

Other uses of *Helianthus annus*
Its residue is used as fodder for cattle and manure.

Other hazards of *Helianthus annus*
Some people are allergic to sunflower foliage and may react with a skin rash.

Cucumis sativus Linn.

Cucumis sativus is known by kakra in Nepali language and saret in Lepcha language. It belongs to the family Cucurbitaceae. It is a creeping vine that bears cylindrical fruits that are used as culinary vegetables. It is cultivated all over Sikkim and Darjeeling hills.

Parts used for medicine
Fruit & seeds

Medicinal uses
The fruit has carminative and antacid properties. The leaf juice is emetic and it is used to treat dyspepsia in children. The fruit is depurative, diuretic, emollient, purgative and resolvent. The fresh fruit is used internally in the treatment of blemished skin, heat rash etc. It is also used externally as a poultice for burns, sores etc and also as a cosmetic for softening the skin. The seed is a cooling, diuretic, tonic and vermifuge. One grams of thoroughly ground seeds (including the seed coat) is used to expel the worms from the body. A decoction of the root is diuretic. Fruits and seeds have cooling, nutritious property and promote urination in painful passage of urine and suppression of urine.

Other uses of *Cucumis sativus*
Eaten raw in form of salad or prickles.

Other hazards of *Cucumis sativus*
Not yet known.

Curcuma aromatic Salish.

Curcuma aromatic is known by hardi in Nepali language and salek in Lepcha language. It is a perennial herb belongs to the family Zingiberaceae. It grows wild throughout Sikkim and Darjeeling hills.

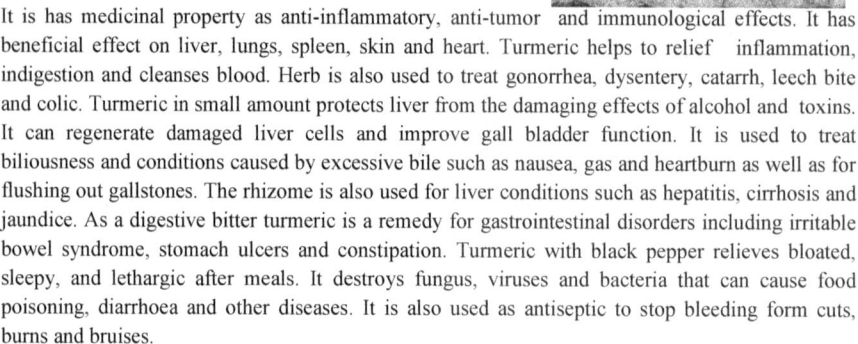

Parts used for medicine
Rhizome

Medicinal uses
It is has medicinal property as anti-inflammatory, anti-tumor and immunological effects. It has beneficial effect on liver, lungs, spleen, skin and heart. Turmeric helps to relief inflammation, indigestion and cleanses blood. Herb is also used to treat gonorrhea, dysentery, catarrh, leech bite and colic. Turmeric in small amount protects liver from the damaging effects of alcohol and toxins. It can regenerate damaged liver cells and improve gall bladder function. It is used to treat biliousness and conditions caused by excessive bile such as nausea, gas and heartburn as well as for flushing out gallstones. The rhizome is also used for liver conditions such as hepatitis, cirrhosis and jaundice. As a digestive bitter turmeric is a remedy for gastrointestinal disorders including irritable bowel syndrome, stomach ulcers and constipation. Turmeric with black pepper relieves bloated, sleepy, and lethargic after meals. It destroys fungus, viruses and bacteria that can cause food poisoning, diarrhoea and other diseases. It is also used as antiseptic to stop bleeding form cuts, burns and bruises.

Other uses of *Curcuma aromatic*
Used as spices.

Other hazards of *Curcuma aromatic*
Do not use turmeric if you have gallstones or a bile duct obstruction. Taking turmeric might slow blood clotting. This might increase the risk of bruising and bleeding in people with bleeding disorders. It might decrease blood sugar in people with diabetes.

Cydonia oblonga Will.

Cydonia oblonga is known by sahaor paot in Lepcha language. It belongs to the family Rosaceae. It grows wild in the forest of lower and mid hill of Sikkim and Darjeeling.

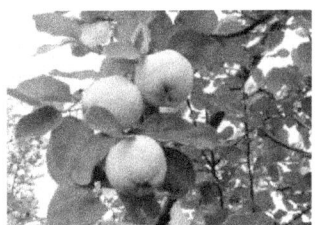

Parts used for medicine
Fruits
Medicinal uses
Fruits are pounded into paste and smeared over the forehead for curing headache. The cooked fruit helps to stimulate the heart in cases of heart failure. It is also good for treating digestive disorders and gastrointestinal inflammation. It is also used as a poultice for injuries, inflammation of the joints, injuries of the nipples and gashed or deeply cut fingers.

Other uses of *Cydonia oblonga*
It is used to make jam, jelly and quince pudding. The fruit can be eaten in the raw as well as cooked form.

Other hazards of *Cydonia oblonga*
Prolonged use or excess internal doses might lead to gastric irritation.

Evodia fraxinifolia Hook.

Evodia fraxinifolia is known by khanakpa in Nepali language and kanu in Lepcha language. It belongs to the family Rutaceae. It is fodder tree which grows up to an altitude of 4000 to 8000 ft. and attains the height of 50 ft.

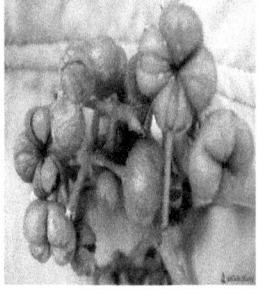

Parts used for medicine
Fruit and whole plant.

Medicinal uses
The plant is antipyretic and used in the treatment of typhoid. It has diuretic properties. Fruits are used in the treatment of indigestion.

Other uses of *Evodia fraxinifolia*
Not yet known.
Other hazards of *Evodia fraxinifolia*
Not yet known.

Abies webbiana Lind.

Abies webbiana is known by ghurbis in Nepali language and daong sying koong in Lepcha language. It belongs to the family Rutaceae. It is straight growing tree widely distributed in temperate and sub-alpine Himalayas of Darjeeling and Sikkim at an altitude ranges from 5200-13800 ft.

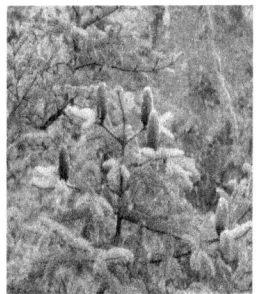

Parts used for medicine
Leaves and gums

Medicinal uses
Leaves are carminative, expectorant, stomachic, tonic astringent. It is a tonic and used in hoarse voice, internal haemorrhage and tuberculosis. The gum mixed with oil of rose when taken internally helps in intoxication and externally used against headache and neuralgia. Leaves mixed with ginger, cardamom, cloves and sugar is used for asthma and bronchitis .Oil extracted from the leaves is used in hoarseness, internal haemorrhage and tuberculosis.

Other uses of *Abies webbiana*
Ink can be prepared from after boiling.
Other hazards of *Abies webbiana*
Not yet known.

Viscum album Linn.

Viscum album is known by harchur in Nepali language and sun tee pro in Lepcha language. It belongs to the family Loranthaceae. It is a semi- parasitic evergreen shrub found on branches of trees in the forests of mid and upper hill of Sikkim and Darjeeling.

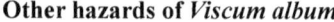

Parts used for medicine
Whole plant.

Medicinal uses
The herb is bitter, acrid, cooling, sweetish, alexipharmic, aphrodisiac, alternative and useful in "Kapha" and "Vata", diseases of blood, ulcers, epilepsy, biliousness. Whole plant is used as a poultice for treatment of muscular pain and also in case of fracture. A decoction of plant is also given in aching limbs. It is also resolvent and laxative. In the hills it is used in treating muscular pains, injuries and fractures and also in decoction in fever with aching limbs.

Other hazards of *Viscum album*
Not yet known.
Other uses of *Viscum album*
Not yet known.

Schima wallichii Choisy.

Schima wallichii is known by chilauney in Nepali language and sungbraang koong in Lepcha language. It belongs to the family Theaceae. *S. Wallichii* is an evergreen tree found abundantly in temperate and sub tropical climate in the forests of lower and mid hill of Sikkim and Darjeeling.

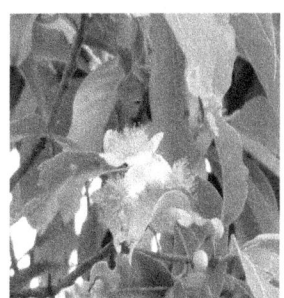

Parts used for medicine
Bark, leaves and roots

Medicinal uses
The young plants, leaves and roots are used for the treatment of fevers. The bark is anthelmintic and rubefacient. Bark juice is given to animals infested with liver flukes. Fruit pulp is an antidote against scorpion bites. Bark is irritant and vermicide and is used for curing gonorrhoea.

Other uses of *Schima wallichii*
Use as fodder, mulching materials, fuel and timber.

Other hazards of *Schima wallichii*
Not yet known.

Cinnamomum tamala (Buch.-Ham.) T.Nees & C.H.Eberm.

Cinnamomum tamala is known by Tejpata in Nepali language and also known as tejapatta, Malabar leaf, Indian bark, Indian cassia. It belongs to the family Lauraceae. It grows up to 20 m tall. It has aromatic leaves which are used for culinary and medicinal purposes. It is an evergreen tree found abundantly in temperate and sub tropical climate in the forests of lower and mid hill of Sikkim and Darjeeling.

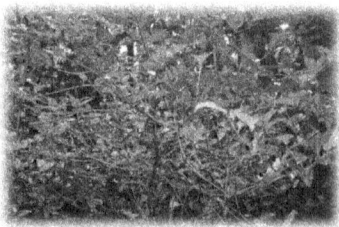

Parts used for medicine
Bark and leaves

Medicinal uses
The bark is aromatic and given in gonorrhoea. Leaves are stimulant and carminative and used in rheumatism, colic, reduction in blood glucose level, blood glycosylated haemoglobin, therapy in diabetes and diarrhoea.

Other hazards of *Cinnamomum tamala*
Not yet known.

Other uses of *Cinnamomum tamala*
Culinary purposes

Ficus cunia Buch.-Ham. ex Roxb.

It is a tree with a flat, spreading, umbrella-like crown; it grows up to 3 - 10 metres tall and bole may be 15 - 25cm in diameter. It grows wild in the forests and river valleys of lower hills of Sikkim and Darjeeling.

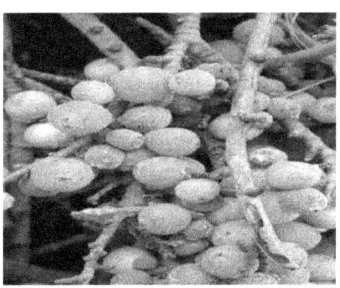

The tree is gathered from the wild for its edible fruit, fibre and medicinal properties. It is also cultivated as a shade tree along the sides of roads. It belongs to the family Moraceae

Parts used for medicine
Roots and fruits.

Medicinal uses
Fruit juice if taken regularly and the affected parts if washed with it cure leprosy. Juice of the roots and bark cooked in milk cures bladder complaints.

Other hazards of *Ficus cunia*
Not yet known.
Other uses of *Ficus cunia*
Not yet known.

Selected references

1. Anonymous, 1948-1976. The wealth of India- a dictionary of Indian raw material and natural products,Vols.I-II,CSIR,New Delhi.
2. Bodding,P.O.(Rv.),1925.Studies in santal medicines and connected folklore.Part I & II.Mern.Asiatic Society Bengal.10:1-427
3. Chopra,R.N.,Nayar,S.L., and Chopra,I.C.(1958).Glossary of Indian medicinal plants.CSIR,New Delhi.
4. Jain,S.K.(1971). Medicinal Plants. National Book Trust,New Delhi.
5. Maheshwari, P. and Singh,U. (1964). Dictionary of economic plants of India.ICRI,New Delhi.

www.ingramcontent.com/pod-product-compliance
Lightning Source LLC
Chambersburg PA
CBHW060408190526
45169CB00002B/810